Praise for *Plu*

"This book will change your life and your yoga practice. It is raw, real, exposed, vulnerable, and straight to the heart. As a yoga teacher and a mother and general life seeker, I find Cori's personal story to fill me with inspiration, revelation and a desire to keep walking the path." – Peach Friedman-Dumars, Author of *Diary of an Exercise Addict*

"I found myself unexpectedly sinking in. From family to business, from practice to teaching, this book shares insights, tragedies, victories and revivals of mind, body and spirit. Cori is honest, makes space for our reality and inquiry, and reminds us of the divinity in everything. Plus One is a great read - it's fun and deep and just feels right." – Elena Brower, Author of *Art of Attention*

"A must read for anyone who has struggled with their own critical inner voice." – Jennifer Marrero, MA, NCC, LPC

Praise for *Plus One* (cont.)

"Cori writes from a place that radiates truth, freedom and love. Dive into each page as if she was speaking directly to you because on a soul level, she is."
- Dana Damara, Author of Om's From the Mat

"Cori Martinez courageously chronicles her journey as a yoga professional with vulnerability, tenderness and fierce honesty. The result is a captivating story that will inspire you to live life with bravery and an open heart."
- Amy Ippoliti, yoga teacher and co-founder of 90 Monkeys

Plus One

Finding God on the Yoga Mat

By Cori Martinez

Marlo Books, Sebastopol, CA

Marlo Books, Sebastopol CA
PO Box 225, Sebastopol, CA. 95473
© 2013 by Cori Martinez

2013
USA
978-0-615-91632-3
Paper durability statement—This paper meets the
requirements of ANSI/NISO Z39.48-1992

For Kalia

Your presence in my life changed everything. From
the moment you were born, (actually, from my second
day of contractions) you asked more of me than I ever
thought I could give and showed me how good it feels
to say yes. You gave me a reason to long for a higher
power. You broke my heart wide open and showed me
just how deeply I could love. May our life together
be happy, healthy and filled with loving-kindness
and peace. May you always love yourself as much as
I love you, sweet girl.

A Gift From Danna Faulds

"Walk Slowly"

It only takes a reminder to breathe,
a moment to be still, and just like that,
something in me settles, softens, makes
space for imperfection. The harsh voice
of judgment drops to a whisper and I
remember again that life isn't a relay
race; that we will all cross the finish
line; that waking up to life is what we
were born for. As many times as I
forget, catch myself charging forward
without even knowing where I'm going,
that many times I can make the choice
to stop, to breathe, and be, and walk
slowly into the mystery.

Contents

Gratitude

Authors and teachers: Claire Derderer, it was after reading *Poser* that I was first inspired to write this book. Natalie Goldberg, it was *Old Friend from Far Away* that helped me to put words on a page. Mark Nepo, your words in *Exquisite Risk* inspired me as I wrote and your words from many places hold true in my heart and soul. Byron Katie, who surely does not need my gratitude, you have it eternally. Thank you, Katie, for asking me (whenever it hurts) if what I'm believing is true and for giving me the space to see for myself that it's not. It is The Work you share that continuously breaks down barriers in my mind so that I may truly know God in myself, and all beings.

To my yoga students past and present: For 15 years you have shown up to listen and consider what I have to say, leaving me to finally believe I have something worthwhile to offer. Thank you for showing up, for the gratitude you've shared, the insights you've offered, the dedication you've shown, and the extreme inspiration you've provided. I still think of so many of you from Yoga Centered; know that you will always be in my heart.

Asha Yoga and Yoga Centered teachers, staff and karma yogi's: Your work has made it possible for me to live my dream life. Thank you for helping me create a warm, welcoming environment for a community of yogis to safely unwind and discover the best version of themselves.

My friends: Jennifer Marrero and Kaitlin Mundle, thanks for cheering me on when I announced from my hammock in Mexico that I wanted to write a book. And Jennifer, thank you for counseling me through leading my first Yoga Teacher Training and giving me the strength and courage to keep learning and growing. Without you I may not have discovered my passionate love for teaching teachers. Emily Epstein, thank you for so much, but in particular, for Old Turtle. You knew I could barely speak the word God and you showed me gently (and with beautiful art) a way of seeing God and sharing this spirit with my daughter. Reading this book aloud to her was the first time I spoke the word in a loving way. Chantill Lopez, thank you for walking with me hand-in-hand for 15 years, I am at a loss for any other words. I love you, Chantill. I love you all, even if I never remember your birthdays!

To my mother-in-law, Becky Martinez, who has treated me like her own flesh and blood for as long as I can remember. Thank you, Becky, for showing me a version of family I didn't know, with homemade cookies and cakes and pies, and tables set with linens and crystal and candles. Thank you for coming to the rescue again and again, so often without needing to be asked, and for too many more things to list here. Most of all, thank you for raising a son who is both tremendously strong and incredibly loving, who is an amazing father, husband, and life partner.

My Dad, Jim Kozlovich: Thank you, Dad, for respecting my beliefs and views, so different from yours, to make room for discovering our similarities. Thank you for trusting me when I asked you to, and making it possible for me to build Asha Yoga. Thank you so very much for giving your blessing that I write in these pages what feels true for me, from my perspective.

Mom: Thank you for loving me the way I love my own daughter, even when I was (and still am) a pain-in-the-ass. Thank you for wanting so much and working so hard to make my childhood better than yours...and for succeeding a million times over. Though you may never believe me, I promise you in print, I am very, very grateful.

Josh Martinez, my husband and best friend: Thank you for loving me for almost half of my life. Thank you for taking care of me when I need it, for putting up with me when I am totally self-absorbed, and for believing in me and pushing me to be better than I sometimes think I can be. And thank you, thank you, thank you, for being the best father our daughter could ask for. I love you, babe.

P.S. Thank you, Yon Walls, for telling me I had started something great with this book and tugging at me to keep on writing; Catherine Escobedo and Emily Taggart for diving in wholeheartedly and handing me a brilliantly edited final copy I am so proud of; and Anita Claypatch for the beautiful design.

Cori Martinez

Introduction

"In your light I learn how to love. In your beauty, how to make poems. You dance inside my chest where no-one sees you, but sometimes I do, and that sight becomes this art."

– Rumi

Once upon a time ago, my effort to be recognized, approved of and admired was illuminated and reflected back to me in a Bikram Yoga studio mirror. Although my practice evolved beyond Bikram Yoga, that evolving practice continued to reveal what was

7

deep inside of me. Revelation after revelation, layer by layer, as I unfolded on my mat, I finally had to consider that I had landed in a spiritual practice. Even if all I had wanted was an easy "A" and a cuter body.

Yoga is a Sanskrit word that means "Union with God." Most people think yoga is a physical practice about stretching and strengthening the body, not realizing that what we call yoga is what history calls asana. Asana is only one part of yoga and yoga is actually defined as an experience of uniting with God. The most popular form of yoga in the United States and Europe today is the kind where you use the physical body as a vehicle to connect with God.

15 million people are practicing this physical yoga today because it does more than get our body in shape. It invites us into the perspective that everything is Sacred: every emotion, apparent flaw, sensation, action, reaction, loss, gain, success, failure, birth, death, animal and tree. All things are worthy; all things are Sacred.

At its core, yoga invites us to see God everywhere. To say yes and trust in the unfolding of life, to be willing to let go of our stories and attachments in exchange for unmistakable divinity in all things, including ourselves.

Plus One is a memoir of spiritual life sneaking up on me and the story of how my practice of yoga and conscious living led to an unexpected meeting and deep friendship with both humanity and God. When I began to practice yoga, I wasn't looking for this kind of connection. My intentions were far less altruistic. Yet, year after year I unrolled my mat to move and breathe and pay attention until one day I found myself in this deep friendship. I found that what I had come to believe in, what I had come to trust without a doubt, brought me a peace I had never even known was there to want. Because of this connection, I fall in love with life again and again, often unconditionally, and that is what I wish for you and all of humanity.

Through my story, it is my great hope to inspire in you an intimate connection with the life you are living, to ignite reverence for your humanness and to instill trust in the divinity of all things.

Cori Martinez

In that,

May you fall in love with your life unconditionally
and
find each and every moment to be
so much more than enough.

Practice

When I step onto my yoga mat. I feel my feet sink in and somehow connect with the ground beneath the floorboards. I turn inward and deepen my breath, opening to a vibrancy that radiates from below my skin, far out beyond the perimeter of my physical body. Just by standing, turning inward and breathing, I am lightly caressed by a thousand invisible fingers. My body responds by softening. My low back, neck, shoulders, jaw, and eyes let go slightly and their need to control begins to dissolve.

My need to control begins to dissolve.

Cori Martinez

I reach my arms up overhead, farther and farther, spreading my fingers until there is new space between my ribs and between my ribcage and pelvis. My collarbones widen as my shoulders inch back. My heart is opening. My eyes lift up and I am full of breath, yes, but also much more. I am awake, inspired, spacious. I pause.

On an exhale, I bow down, folding at the crease at the top of my thighs, and surrender to the day just as it is. I empty my breath completely to make room for the overwhelming gratitude that rushes in. I close my eyes. It feels so good to move, to open, to feel.

In the first forward fold, my knees bend slightly, but as my hamstrings gradually warm with each repetition, my legs eventually pull straight, lift up and press back. Rooting through the center of my heels, I inhale and lift halfway back up, with an emphasis on physically opening across my chest and filling my whole torso again with breath. I exhale and bow forward again, relaxing my neck and letting the crown of my head sink toward the earth.

This is asana. In the 21st century it entails stepping onto a rubber mat, moving, breathing and pausing. We call it yoga. Approximately 2000 years ago asana was listed as one of eight things one must do to experience yoga, then defined as "Union with God," resulting in wholeness and inner peace.

As I bow down once again, touching my fingers to the ground, I am offered this gift long before I know I want it.

I leave the studio. Everywhere I go I say, "Hello"—to Stan in the surf shop, to George-the-Cashier at Abundant Life, to Keith at the farmers market, to Rick and Peggy at the t-shirt printing shop, to people everywhere in yoga clothes, carrying yoga mats, on their way to or coming from class at Yoga Centered.

One day George-the-Cashier tells me, "You know, you changed this town. You, with all your smiling and your yoga. It's been very amazing to watch."

I smile.

Inside, I'm feeling both pride and discomfort.

Cori Martinez

The Dream Life

"She looked around and saw that
life was pretty amazing."

– Unknown

My mom and Bob fell in love within 24 hours, moved in together after a week and were married six months after that. Bob lived in Hawaii for 13 years and had just sold his helicopter company before moving back to California when he met my mom. Not long after they were married, he began missing the ocean air and the palm trees. He wanted to move back to Hawaii and had the idea to start a mushroom farm. Josh and I had graduated college and were still waiting tables and bartending. When they proposed a partnership, we jumped on board. Neither of us had ever dreamed of living in Hawaii the way some people do, but when the idea surfaced...we began to.

We shipped a houseful of furniture, both of our vehicles and everything else we owned to the Big Island of Hawaii without even seeing it first. We were full of hope, trust and adventure with big plans to start a commercial mushroom farm with my Mom and her new husband, Bob.

The first month, it rained 36 inches, which is A LOT. We read to expect 10-15 inches of rain per month in Hilo, the wettest city in the world. At first it rains all the time and we wonder...*What have we done?* Then the sun comes out and our new life in Hawaii is amazing.

Josh is driving, and whoever is visiting is in the back seat. The sky is light blue and white and the sun rests on the water. Or it's pouring down rain so hard we might have to pull over and wait. It still rains a lot.

We're on our way to the beach, or to a waterfall, or a tide pool. Maybe to the warm ponds, where steam vents from the lava flowing below open up into the bottom of salt water pools, naturally making the water about 90 degrees. We'll find sun somewhere. We've learned it's never far.

There are towels in the trunk with one ice chest full of food and another filled with beer. There's a rainbow and the smell of gardenias, plumerias and salt water.

Cardinals are in the parking lots; feral cats are everywhere. Flying termites and cockroaches no longer send me screaming.

After the beach we dust black sand, or white, or maybe green sand from our feet, if we came from the beach where the waves crash against the lava filled with green crystals.

We cook dinner. Or go for Thai food at Naung Mai. I order spring rolls with a side of large green leaves of lettuce, mint, cucumbers, and sweet chili dip. I wrap the lettuce around the crispy fried spring rolls and pile the mint and cucumbers inside.

We drink mai tais. Josh makes the mix from scratch. We find *lilikoi*, passion fruit, on a vine by the waterfall, guava from a neighbor's tree, fresh pineapple juice, and sometimes we squeeze fresh oranges. It's $4 for an orange. It's $8 for hummus. (I return the $7 yellow bell pepper.)

Our best friends moved to Hawaii with us. Sometimes they live with us. Sometimes they have their own ocean view apartment on the side of the highway. Once a cockroach crawls into Carlos's ear and twice Josh gets bitten by a centipede. The flying termites swarm our kitchen if we turn the lights on at night so we cook in the dark, or by candlelight. We don't have curtains so we wake up with the sun—and the neighbor's rooster.

This is life our first six months in Hawaii. We are living our honeymoon, even though we aren't married yet.

The Ocean

"For each of us is like a great untamed sea, obedient
to deeper currents that are seldom visible."

– Mark Nepo

I think the ocean was the very first thing to show
me the meaning of union, wholeness and inner peace.
I have loved the ocean for as long as I can remember.
Although I had always felt it deeply, I didn't know
how to explain the sense I had of two bodies of salt
water—mine and the vast Pacific's—seeming to be part
of the same whole. When I see the ocean move with

grace and ease, even in the midst of a massive storm, I know I have the same capacity.

Living at the edge of the sea, I want to learn to surf. My student and friend, Summer, takes me out to the Hilo surf spot, Honolii. It is less than half a mile from the yoga studio and it is not a hip trendy beach with girls in Brazilian bikinis. There's no surfboard rental shack or an option to purchase a lesson or ride tandem on some big giant board the size of a boat that would be nearly impossible to fall off of. There's black sand, rocks on the floor of the ocean, and salt water as far as I can see. The water is filled with locals. Even though I spend 80 percent of my life in Hawaii barefoot and the other 20 percent in flip-flops, I step timidly over the rocks, secretly wincing from the sharp edges.

I'm not afraid of a shark attack, even though the news has recently been obsessed with shark attacks, to the point it seems from the reporting to be highly likely I'll be eaten alive. The obsession and exaggeration of the danger makes me defensive of my current home state. I research to find that from 1828 to January 2005 there have only been a total of 98 unprovoked shark attacks in Hawaii, only eight of which were fatal. Getting in a car accident on the way to the beach is a much greater possibility than being attacked by a shark, so I'm not worried.

I want to commune with the ocean, to be one with this mysterious and beautiful body that endlessly continues to flow with grace and ease under any circumstance. But I'm cold. Plus, I have a terrible sense of direction. So when Summer tells me about a large rock just under the surface of the water that I have to always be aware of and avoid, my vision of being a surfer immediately begins to blur.

At this point I am teaching about 10 yoga classes per week and practicing on my own. I've had "yoga photos" taken recently, the kind yoga teachers take for promotional purposes, showing off our apparently desirable skills in crazy arm balances and headstands. When I look at these pictures I'm impressed by the defined muscles in my arms, my shoulders, and my back. I am strong. Yet, here I am in the water trying to surf and—with purple lips, teeth chattering and goose bumps everywhere—I thrash almost uselessly at the unresponsive salty mass around me. Getting the surfboard out far enough to wait for a wave is hard, but then swimming fast enough to actually catch one seems nearly impossible. My favorite part is when the water swells enough to make the board and me both weightless for a moment, and there is no catchable wave in sight. Then, I am truly at peace.

As soon as a potential wave emerges, Summer tells me to get on my belly and at the sound of her command, "GO. Swim hard and fast."

Rarely can I swim fast enough. Sometimes I miss the break completely. Sometimes I catch it just enough to be tossed off my board, pummeled roughly into the water and tumbled senselessly like a ragdoll. *How in the world am I supposed to keep track of the giant rock????* I cover my head with my arms and squeeze my eyes as tightly as possible, obviously holding my breath.

On the rare occasion when I do catch the wave and ride it all the way to shore on my belly—or a few times squatting on my board—my excitement is stunted by the realization that I am going to have to repeat all this. I'll have to walk on the rocks again, paddle all the way back out again, hope to ride a wave again.

After a week or two, I stand on shore holding a surfboard for the last time and gaze longingly at the single outcast in the water—the only surfer wearing a full body wetsuit and a helmet. If only I had the courage to show up in a wetsuit and a helmet, I might have a fighting chance of learning to surf. But no, that would be far too condemnable.

So instead, I quit.

Cori Martinez

Meeting Yoga

"Practice and all is coming."
– Sri K. Pattabhi Jois

Psychology of Hatha Yoga was a four-unit class and we were allowed to take it twice for credit. When people ask me how I got into yoga, my honest answer is, "It seemed like an easy 'A.'" And I did get an "A." Both times. Because the first time I cheated on the final, a Karma Yoga project.

Karma is the law of cause and effect. Karma Yoga is basically about doing good stuff so that good stuff comes back to you. I kept intending to start my project, but the week before it was due I found myself borrowing my friend's five-year-old daughter so I could take pictures of her in yoga poses and claim that I had been teaching her yoga for months.

I have a picture of her balancing on one leg in Tree Pose and another doing Lion's Breath—her tongue out, mouth and eyes wide. As I pass the glossy 4x5 pictures around my class circle, I tell my classmates that her mom had needed a babysitter so I had agreed to watch her free of charge and teach her yoga.

While still in college I take my first Bikram Yoga class, which I love from the very first moment. I love the heat, the sweat, and the teacher saying my name, "Beautiful arch, Cori." "Very nice, Cori," she would say. I push a little harder when I hear my name, though I try to appear calm and serene.

There are mirrors lining the walls.

I look at myself in the mirror: *young, thin, flexible, strong.* I smile knowing the teacher has noticed. Then she would say, "Beautiful opening, Jennifer," or, "Very good, Jim," and I want to hear my own name again.

What about me? I look at the teacher, so cute in her stretchy black shorts and tiny little top . . .

She has a strong curvy body. I look back again at myself in the mirror. I look different now. My legs are too skinny. My nose is too big. My skin is too white. I push harder. I can do it. My friend Karen can do it. I check out of the corner of my eye. I watch her until I fold forward and the sweat pours out of my body, pools into my eyes and temporarily blinds me.

It's hot. 109-degrees hot. I straighten my leg, lock it out, round my back and reach my forehead to my knee. It touches. The teacher notices. "Yes, Cori! Just like that! Good!"

I think: *I need some super-short shorts and a black bra top. I might throw up. No, I might faint. It. Is. Hot.* I put my foot down and smile ever so slightly at my blurry, wet image in the mirror.

In Hawaii I begin to daydream about a vibrant yoga community in Hilo, about building that community myself and living the life of a yoga teacher. My mom has been self-employed my entire life. My dad too. And Josh's parents. The possibility of failure doesn't even occur to me. Six months after moving to Hawaii we buy a house and I fly to Houston to complete a Yoga Teacher Training.

I think no one in this training believes I will become a yoga teacher. I am lost every time I try to teach a pose. The fear of saying the wrong thing paralyzes me from being able to say anything and I literally cannot get a single word out. I laugh nervously and smile a lot. At night in my hotel room my new friends urge me gently, "Just say anything. You know the poses. Something is better than nothing. You can do it." I don't tell them I'm planning to teach as soon as the training's over. I'm afraid of anyone thinking I believe I can do it when they think I can't. That somehow feels even more humiliating.

But on the last day of the training, I teach Shoulder Stand to the entire room for our final exam. I am calm, clear, and casually charismatic. Although I imagine everyone else is shocked, I notice I don't feel entirely surprised. I feel like I always knew I could do it, but didn't want anyone else to know, just in case. It's safer this way, believing I don't have far to fall in the eyes of everyone watching. I don't notice yet how much more afraid I am of being perceived as a failure than of actually failing.

Before opening my first yoga studio, Yoga Centered, I start renting space by the hour and teaching a few classes at various places around town: a massage studio, a macadamia nut factory, a gym, and then I find this place above the farmers market. The entrance is in an alley and there's no address. Up two flights of narrow, winding, wooden stairs, that would no way in the world ever pass building code in California, there's a tiny little bathroom. Up one more flight is a door to a dirty room with peeling, faded, Pepto-Bismol-pink paint on the walls, broken window shades and splintery-raw wood floors. I pace the room and guess (correctly) that twelve mats could fit. The back corner of the room has been walled off to make a very tiny office or storage space. I'm looking for another location to rent by the hour. This might work if I can get a good deal and am willing to do some heavy duty cleaning.

"Why don't you just rent it month-to-month?" the guy says.

"Oh. Well. I can't. I can't afford to do that."

"I'll give you a good deal," he says.

"What kind of good deal?"

"No rent while you clean it up a bit. Then how about $500 a month?"

"How about $400?" I say. "Including utilities."

"OK, sure, sounds good."

Eleven days later, I have a sign, sage-green walls, bamboo rolling shades, a self-sanded and lacquered wood floor, a cute little bathroom, and an ad in the local alternative paper. I really didn't know I was going to open a yoga studio until I was standing in the finished space. It was perfect.

My home phone begins to ring. I have to do a lot of explaining about what yoga is and who it's for. "Everyone," I say. "No, not just hippies." "No, we won't do anything weird." And of course: "Yes, it's OK if you can't touch your toes."

People begin to show up for classes. Within a month, 12 people are showing up for some of the classes—the exact maximum that could fit if the mats were placed just perfectly staggered. After two months

I decide to get rid of the office in order to fit more mats. In one long day, Josh and I demo the walls, patch the floors and paint. At the end of the day, 17 mats can fit. And IN THE VERY NEXT CLASS, 17 bodies show up to unroll their mats and practice.

Students sign in by marking their 3x5 index card, color-coded based on the type of pass they buy, from the box where they're alphabetized by first name.

I am teaching 18 classes a week, until I hire my first teacher, Heather. She's new to Hilo, funny, smart, extremely charismatic, passionate about yoga and . . . *maybe a little younger than me?* We become fast friends.

A week before I'm planning to leave for my first vacation since opening the studio six months before, Heather wants to meet. She's going to be subbing all my classes while I'm gone. I am nervous, but I trust her.

When we meet she tells me that she's been doing some calculations. She's looked through the card box and added up how much money I'm collecting per student for each class. Since 'her classes are bringing in that amount multiplied by the number of students who show up for her class, she feels she should get that amount when she teaches.' In other words, it seems fair to her that she keeps 100 percent of what the students are paying to attend her class, even though I'm the one who answers the phone in my house, returns messages, and pays for the rent, the upkeep, the ad in the paper, the flyers, the insurance, and the yoga mats (because no one owns their own yoga mat yet). Even though I'm the one that papers the town with flyers and teaches free classes at community events to get people in the door, she feels she is bringing in the people if they are in her class.

I think she's crazy.

And I have no idea that this is only the beginning of a long debate between me, as a studio owner, and the next 100 yoga teachers I will hire throughout my career.

Heather says she understands. However, there's a new studio opening around the corner and that owner is offering to pay her 100 percent of what each student pays to attend her class. It's a deal she can't pass up, so I could either match it or she'll move on.

I go home and cry.

I'm afraid of competition, of losing students, of losing my only other teacher and taking on more classes again.

I'm defensive about the perception that it's easy to get people to show up, that I'm raking in a bunch of cash and keeping it all for myself.

I'm angry that she looked through the card box and calculated the money coming in (first, without calculating the money or time going out, and second, for doing it at all).

I'm hurt that someone I thought was a friend would be so matter-of-fact about leaving.

We agree that Heather would move on, but after I got back from my trip. She would still sub for all of my classes.

When I come back, a student tells me that Heather posted flyers for the new studio on our bulletin board and handed out her schedule while I was gone. Heather doesn't deny this; she simply doesn't see anything wrong with it.

We talk it out, and in the end she apologizes. I say I understand. We hug and say goodbye, wishing each other well. I think she may have been sincere, but I know that as much as I want to be, I am not. Eventually Heather takes over the new studio and we become the owners of the only two yoga studios in town for the next seven years. For seven years I pretend everything is fine between us, but deep down I remain hurt and angry.

Soon after Heather leaves my studio—about nine months after opening Yoga Centered in the alley—I'm downtown and I look through the storefront windows of a beautiful large building that used to be a bank. It is raw and empty with nothing but concrete inside. I get the keys a few days later and begin overseeing construction to transform the empty space into a yoga studio and boutique.

At this point, I am no stranger to construction. Already, since living in Hawaii, we have bought and majorly renovated a house and built a 20,000 square foot indoor mushroom farm with my mom and Bob, in addition to fixing up the first yoga studio.

Something I always forget, but am reminded of each time I've opened a studio, is that the build out period is CRAZY BUSY. The phone never stops ringing, there are endless schedules to organize, numbers to crunch, and decisions to make and re-make (and re-make again) when each step doesn't turn out quite the way someone anticipated. There are business cards to design and order, signs to print, websites to build, employees to hire, insurance policies to adjust or create, and Federal ID numbers, business licenses, and permits to get, and on and on and on. If you already have a business, you must do all of this at the same time that you're operating your current location(s). This is when I get my very first cell phone and experience the addictive convenience most of the world will soon come to depend on.

After I sign the lease, my little brother comes to visit. We are standing in the still raw space, concrete dust everywhere, and I'm telling him all about what it's going to look like: 14-feet long, deep dark-green curtains, wood floors, pale-gold walls, and dark reddish-brown columns. The front desk is already being built. While I'm talking to my brother, an ambulance drives by with its sirens blaring. Loudly. I actually roll my eyes. (This is a story I didn't admit to for a very long time.)

"Well, that's going to be just great during a final relaxation pose!" I say.

My little brother looks at me in confusion. He is 18 and has never done any yoga. Then he says,

"That doesn't seem very yogic. Shouldn't you be, like, happy or something that someone in need is getting some help? Or compassionate for someone who's in trouble? Instead of worried about the noise of the siren?"

"Oh . . . right," I mumble, embarrassed that hadn't occurred to me.

But the sound of the siren never bothers me again. And to this day, about 15 years later, I thank my brother for showing me that what I practice and teach about is meant to be applied to everything, to expand my automatic perception of life with more consciousness and kindness.

The new space at 37 Waianuenue Avenue can fit 40 people. On opening day, exactly 40 people show up for class and unroll their mats. The fact that this

I

keeps happening cannot be a coincidence. I take it as a sign. I have made the right decision. I feel The Island guiding me every step of the way in this yoga venture, and certainly embracing me. After class, 80 more slip off their shoes at the front door and gather for Hawaiian music and *pupus* (pronounced "poo-poo's"), the Hawaiian word for "snacks or appetizers"— yes, really! Along with shoes and bodies, the studio fills up with flowers. Everyone brings giant bouquets of orchids, Birds of Paradise, anthuriums, heliconia, plus I am covered in leis of plumeria and gardenia.

I look around at the people who surround me and realize, with a mix of pride and humility, all that I have done to build this amazing community.

Cori Martinez

Being a Yoga Teacher
Part One

"You know what I love, sweetheart?
The thoughts that used to send us into deep
depression—these same thoughts, once understood,
send us into laughter."
- Byron Katie

I love yoga. I love teaching yoga. At first, I cover my butt with a sweater every time I leave the yoga studio in tight-fitting pants. After six months, I notice a change. I am out to dinner after teaching a class when it occurs to me that I don't feel uncomfortable at all to be wearing yoga clothing in a restaurant. I realize, I hadn't covered anything with a sweater in a long time.

After the new studio opens, I continue to dive into teaching and everything it entails, which is more than one might expect. There are a lot of rules to being a yoga teacher.

For one, yoga teachers (and anyone who wants to be a good person) should definitely recycle. And if they are feeling rushed while cleaning out the fridge and they throw a glass jar with leftovers into the regular garbage, they should immediately cover it up with other garbage, hope no one sees it, and then feel guilty afterward.

Also, they should be healthy and in good physical shape, although how they look should not be important to them. They should not spend too much time getting ready or looking in the mirror. They should not dye their hair, spend too much money on makeup, or shop in chain department stores. They should never go to Wal-Mart!

They should be friendly, forgiving and considerate

of others and their circumstances. They should never get irritated at other drivers, store clerks, telephone sales people, or anyone, really. (Although cigarette smokers could be the only exception to this rule.)

When driving, they should always stop for someone waiting at a crosswalk to cross the street. If they are in a hurry, they should avoid eye contact until it's too late to stop and then pretend to have just noticed the person a moment too late. They should then appear sorry for not seeing the person sooner (soon enough to stop).

They should always give money to homeless people, especially because they should not care about having their own material wealth. Money should be of very minimal importance to a yoga teacher.

They should be in healthy, loving, satisfying relationships and be skilled at communicating with honesty and patience at all times.

They should eat organic foods only: no white flour, processed foods, sugar, caffeine, or alcohol. They should shop only at health-food stores and always bring their own bags. If they forget them, they should stuff everything they can into their purse and carry the rest out piled in their arms, hoping not to drop anything. (Actually, they should definitely not drop anything because they should be graceful most of the time.)

It is OK to be a vegetarian, but ideal to be a vegan, unless they begin to shrivel away and become tired all the time, then eating grass-fed, free-range, organic meat is the only acceptable option. Under these circumstances, however, they should feel very, very guilty for taking the life of another living being for their own selfish purposes. And they should not need to take vitamins because they should get all the vitamins they need from their whole foods, healthy diet.

They should not watch TV. Especially not shows with violence or high levels of personal drama. They should be grateful for every moment, seemingly good or bad, and see the beauty in each and every life experience.

They should have a daily asana, meditation, and pranayama practice. In fact, they should wake up at five every morning and practice for at least two hours, then wash out their nasal passages with warm salt water using a Neti Pot, drink some warm lemon water and eat some vegan stew for breakfast. Then it's time to prepare their fresh organic salad with dark leafy greens, raw veggies, homegrown sprouted grains, and fermented cabbage for lunch. They should plan to pick up some colorful fresh fruit at the farmers market to make a protein smoothie for dinner.

If they get pregnant and have a life or death craving for deep-fried zucchini and ranch dressing from Hot Dog on a Stick in the mall, they should beg their husband to go inside and get it for them (while they hide in the car because they should not be seen eating such crap).

They should be very organized, because their outer environment is a reflection of their calm and clear mind.

They should not need the love and approval of others to be happy, and they should be fully available to give love and acceptance to everyone in their lives.

They should not put anything in life before their

yoga practice, ever. They should be so passionate about sharing the gift of yoga with the world that they should never charge for teaching it because that would not be true to the spirit of the practice.

At the same time, they should make sure to wear organic cotton clothing, made locally by a small company who donates their profits to charity.

And if this gets complicated because they can't figure out how to buy $95 yoga pants, volunteer teach, shop only at health-food stores, and give their money to the homeless (and, of course, other very important causes), they should just go on for years and years feeling guilty every time someone suggests that charging money, making money, or wanting money is not yogic. The guilt is fine—good actually—because guilt is just a sign that they are not living in accordance with their own deepest values, so the guilt that seems to be eating them alive will actually, eventually, lead them to doing and teaching real yoga and living a truly spiritual life.

These are the tried and true rules for yoga teachers (and all good people, really), which I know with total certainty not to be true. But still, for some reason, I declare them and then I try to follow them. Then I judge others and myself on our inability to live up to my unreasonable expectations. Then I try harder.

Often, I am aware of the ridiculousness, the hypocrisy and the contradiction in these rules.

But even as I laugh at them, I am plagued by them.

Cori Martinez

Secrets

"Peace is the result of retraining your
mind to process life as it is, rather than
as you think it should be."

– Wayne Dyer

My mom has told me my whole life that I have a terrible singing voice. She has reminded me that I am "tone deaf and completely lacking of any musical talent whatsoever" more times than I could even begin to count. This is why I blame her when I get lockjaw the first time I chant.

It is the first workshop I have ever hosted at Yoga Centered. A Chanting Workshop, really? I have no idea why. I don't chant, will never chant, not even Om. It just isn't for me.

I sit with the other students as the workshop leader talks, and the nervous inner dialogue that will prove to be there each time I host a workshop for the next several years begins to question:

Will the teacher live up to my expectations? To the students' hopes? Will she accurately represent the studio? Are people going to find value in what she offers? Did I set the expectations too high? How will what she says reflect upon me? Will she say anything that vehemently contradicts what I say when I teach?

It's even worse in this case:

Will everyone notice my horrible singing voice? Will they notice my nervousness? I don't want anyone to know I'm nervous. I don't want to appear self-conscious.

But I am.

So, I smile. And when it comes time to chant, I chant. Every time I hear the sound of my voice over others in the room, I am rigid and self-obsessed, desperate to be confident and OK with my voice. I want that so much more than I want a beautiful voice. My vision of a yoga teacher does not require singing talent, but it does require self-love and acceptance. I am therefore a fraud. My jaw is aching. Stiff. And suddenly it won't open.

Finally, I bow for Namaste. I smile my way out of the workshop and go home. The next day my jaw still won't open. I call an acupuncturist. "How did this happen?" he asks me. "I have NO IDEA," I say. The acupuncturist refers students to me all the time; there is no way in the world I would confess. I go in for a treatment every day for a week, meanwhile eating every meal through a straw, and finally it releases.

I don't tell people that I am easily annoyed by my mom and often ungrateful.

I don't tell them I am extremely defensive with Josh, and that most times when he complains about me being messy or not getting something done, I will spout out a list of things I do and another list of things he doesn't do, and conclude with a statement about how unappreciative, unaccepting, and judgmental he is.

I don't tell anyone that sometimes I scream at the top of my lungs at him and slam the door. I don't share that sometimes I cry so uncontrollably in the midst of these fights—blaming him and then blaming myself—that I have to sleep with tea bags, or cucumbers, or bags of ice on my eyes.

I don't tell people I am 24 years old, because then they might assume I am more of a mess than I let on.

I tell my friends, but I don't tell students, which is totally appropriate, of course. Except...sometimes the voice of shame speaks up, taunting me with the belief that I'm a fraud, that I am entirely flawed, and that if others knew who I really was they would certainly not respect me, or want to learn from me.

At 24, I have created a beautiful community of yogis in a town previously void of yoga. I have already begun to dedicate myself wholeheartedly to what so far appears to be a lifelong mission to share a practice that makes a difference in people's lives. And I am obsessed with being a good person.

Yet so often what drives me is what I'm hiding:

I'm not perfect; I'm not everything I think I should be.

Cori Martinez

Lessons

"Passion will move men beyond themselves, beyond their shortcomings, beyond their failures."

— Joseph Campbell

Even though there is no such thing as social media (no Facebook, Instagram, Twitter, Pinterest, blogs, YouTube, etc.); even though Hawaii residents don't generally look for a website, so ours needs (and gets) no attention from me; I'm not yet a writer, I don't teach teacher trainings and I only have one studio...I am very busy learning.

Because Yoga Centered is a yoga studio and a

boutique, I learn how to run a retail store. I discover along the way what a pre-season order is versus an order "available for immediate delivery." I learn to move product around at least once a week so stuff that's been in the store for a while looks new again. I am getting the hang of Quickbooks, just barely; Josh has to keep reminding me how it works. I spend 80 hours in Publisher and learn to make a black and white, text only, brochure–which I print at the studio and make copies of at the local bookstore around the corner because they also have a copy machine. I make a poster too and then I leave brochures and posters at the surf shops, bookstores, coffee shops, health-food stores, and massage, acupuncture and chiropractic offices. Plus, fifty other places. I do this all myself.

I hire more teachers and a studio manager. Teachers move away and the studio manager goes to nursing school. I hire more teachers again and a new studio manager again. Some version of this happens a few more times and I learn to take the news without freaking out. Twice the iPod is stolen from the studio and I'm totally shocked, both times. Then $1,000 is stolen from the cash drawer and I learn to go to the bank more often.

In addition to running my business, I am also learning my craft. While standing at the front of the room with confidence and charisma comes somewhat natural for me, feeling qualified to teach something does not. So I continue to learn obsessively about the human body and mind as they relate to the system of yoga. I teach between nine and twelve classes a week, which is my favorite part of the day.

Between the mushroom farm and the yoga studio, Josh and I both work a lot. We are either sleeping, at the beach, or working. Mostly, we are working.

I love it. Despite the crazy monkey that lives in my head, jabbering about my imperfections, I love what I do for a living.

I love a student named Aleesha, who came in to try yoga for the first time with a chip on her shoulder and refused to smile. She didn't want to give her last name because she said it was none of our business, so we entered her into the system as Aleesha Aleesha. For the next five years she comes five days a week, and though I never see her smile and I never learn her last name, I do see her soften. And once in a while I see her cry. From Aleesha, I learn the why behind the saying, "Never judge a book by its cover."

I love the regulars who show up faithfully- surfers, construction workers, doctors, nurses, parents, and teenagers. They show up in the midst of divorce, after losing their job, for their bachelorette party, after a night shift, after a funeral, before graduation. They show up and by showing up they teach me about dedication. They are dedicated to something that makes a difference in their lives and even if they can't explain it, they show up. They say thank you. I nod in complete admiration of them.

I learn more and more about the body, about the system of yoga, and about myself.

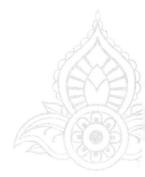

Practice

There are no mirrors. There is no external heat... although since this is Hawaii, there is also no air conditioning.

I move with my breath and music now.

Krishna Das is chanting, even though I never will, and I fold forward to the sound of his devotion.

I inhale and pause to very specifically lengthen the front, side and back of my torso evenly, aligning my ears with my shoulders and reaching through the crown of my head. I check my feet, also very intentionally placed to root through the center of my heels and between the mounds of my toes in order to rebound up through my inner thighs and lift my pelvic floor.

I exhale and get close to my thighs again, drawing my belly button in toward my spine, connecting deeply to the core of my body. I salute the sun, again and again . . . Inhale . . . Upward Facing Dog . . . Exhale . . . Downward Facing Dog . . . Each breath is long, and each movement is placed with detailed care. From Downward Dog I jump through my hands and hover before lowering onto my sitting bones. Just for fun, I lift back up and float back to Chaturanga. Repeat.

I move onto my back to connect even more deeply, more intensely, to my core, not like I'm at the gym. It may look like a cross between a crunch and a sit-up, but it's in slow motion. It may even be on pause. The details of the feet, the inner thighs, the pelvic floor, the low belly, collarbones, neck, jaw, and forehead keep the movement very, very slow. Very effective. Very intense. Yet I am conscious of balancing my effort with ease. The intensity is targeted to avoid my neck and jaw. I place the tip of my tongue softly at the back of my two front teeth where they meet the roof of my mouth to relax my jaw and cradle my head in my hands to relax my neck.

My abs are burning.

I rest before I roll up for Forearm Balance, Handstand, Headstand, backbends galore and then rest again in Pigeon Pose, a Seated Forward Bend, a Reclined Twist, Plow, Fish, and finally, I completely surrender to my mat for Savasana.

Cori Martinez

Mom

"No two persons ever read the same book."

        – Edmund Wilson

I was nine when my dad came into my room and put his face next to mine without even having to lean over. It was one of the only times I have ever seen tears in his eyes.

The frame for my queen-sized mattress was composed of two large dressers and a piece of plywood, making my sleeping quarters about the height of a second story bunk bed, with a fairly spacious secret room below for books and toys and whatever other secret things I wished to store there.

"I'm leaving," he said, "and I'm not coming back." I never saw it coming. But I wouldn't have with my dad. There was no messy divorce battle. He didn't want the house or any money . . . or any visitation rights. In exchange, he wouldn't provide child support.

My mom agreed. She was 32 years old when her 13-year-long marriage came to an end because her husband had fallen madly in love with her own secretary, and she was left alone with their three children ages five, seven, and nine.

I barely saw my dad for almost a year.

My mom, whose own childhood stories are filled with trauma, loss, and abuse, vowed to be the mother she never had. As a single mother, she now had to be good enough that her children would not be scarred by the absence of a father. She worked harder than any mother I will ever know, to succeed at this likely impossible endeavor.

To my brothers, she spoke well of my dad. She protected them with convincing explanations and even untruths: that he called to say goodnight while they were in the bath, or called to say he couldn't make it when he was supposed to pick them up.

It was different with me. I was both the daughter and best friend. Though she will swear forever that she never confessed the truth to me, I know these details because she told them to me.

As a self-employed single mother of three children, she had no time for girlfriends. So as a little girl who loved her mom, I often stepped in. Having me for a friend, however, came at the cost of blurring the delineation between the roles of mother and daughter. She would often shout, "I AM THE MOM!!!" because I would often forget.

When I was 13, we lived in a beautiful custom-built house on our very own hill in Paso Robles, California. We had a sunroom that overlooked a manicured yard with a giant pool surrounded by a forest of oak trees covered in Spanish Moss. We were supposed to have the house for five years, in trade for a design job my mom did for the homeowner. After two years of living peacefully in the beautiful home, the day came when my mom was given a choice: sleep with the homeowner or get out. She refused and suddenly we had no place to live. I didn't realize as we drove away that I would never again share a house with the brothers I had been helping to raise.

My mom and I moved in with Tom and my brothers moved in with our dad. It was supposed to all be temporary. Tom was my mom's friend when she was still married to my dad. He continued to be her friend after the divorce; he once moved in with us and they became more than friends.

My mom wanted to marry him, but he said no. Then he wanted to marry her but she said no. And although that ended their romantic relationship, they are still friends today.

Tom is the one who taught me to drive and helped me buy my first car. When my mom and I moved into his double-wide trailer in a retirement park after getting kicked out of the house on the hill, he was the one who barked at me, "Shut the door behind you," and "Pick up after yourself." For many years, he was the one I called on the third Sunday of June.

Although I never said the words "Happy Father's Day" out of respect for my own father, I called Tom to show my gratitude for all the ways he filled that role.

Although my family's new living arrangement was meant to be temporary, when suddenly my mom was no longer a single mother of three—which had defined her every cell for the past five years—the opportunity to have a completely new identity was a temptation she couldn't resist.

After taking a job in a small beach town 45 minutes away, she fell passionately for a longhaired man who drove a motorcycle and had no children. She rented a tiny studio apartment at the beach and became an unbound single woman in the throes of an irrational love affair.

Half-heartedly, she asked me to move with her to the beach, but after three whole years at the same school for the first time, I desperately did not want to be the new girl again. When the manager of the restaurant I was working at was fired, I lied about my age and got promoted from hostess to full-time floor manager. I applied for work-study at school and swore I could live on my own.

Tom said I could stay with him if I paid rent, although once I proved I could, he never actually made me pay. Sometimes he even offered to match one of my paychecks so I could buy new work or school clothes. Here was another blurry line, this one defining my relationship with Tom. He was part guardian and father figure, yet, while he freely offered his advice, he didn't lay down any rules. I went to school if or when I wanted and I came home at night if or when I wanted, so long as I let him know.

My dad got a job offer in Hawaii and moved there . . . with my brothers. I lived with Tom until I graduated high school. My mom came back once for a few months in the midst of heartbreak, but that is not how she tells the story: She says my brothers needed a little time with their dad and that I was only with Tom for a few months. If you ask her today, she will swear to you it was all only temporary.

I think for a long time she needed to see it as temporary because of how much she needed to believe she was a good mother and, according to her, a good mother would do everything she could to bring us all back together as soon as possible. Eventually, "temporary" became her truth. And since my brothers moved back in with her after she remarried, after seven years of living with our dad, I would concede she has a *case for temporary with my brothers.* I, on the other hand, needed to feel empowered by our separation. I have clung to it my whole life as a way of feeling mature and capable in my relationships and in my business ventures. I have needed to believe that I am mature beyond my years in order to have the confidence to teach women 15 years older than me, in order to hire, manage and fire people sometimes twice my age. I have needed to believe I nearly experienced living on my own and being a grown-up for at least a few years before meeting my husband at the age of 18 so that I won't worry I missed out on something important, I won't feel as though I've never been independent. I *need* everything the way I think it happened to be true. I cannot give my mom her story. And she cannot give me mine. So we go on as two people reading the same book very differently, each of us thinking the other is just a little bit crazy,

as we just barely agree to disagree.

A Baby

"I want to know if you can get up after a night of grief and despair, weary and bruised to the bone, and do what needs to be done for the children."
– Oriah Mountain Dreamer,
The Invitation

When I moved in with Tom, I quit doing drugs, but I did not stop spending the night with boys. Along with my full-time job at the restaurant, I took extra credits at the community college and graduated high school with honors.

I moved away to college with a boy who was five years older than me and we got an apartment. We lived together for two years before I found out he had another girlfriend. He had been seeing her for almost two years.

I got a new apartment and roommate. In college, I repeated my early high school years, with less drugs, more alcohol and no sneaking around. My roommate and I threw parties. We had sleepovers with boys. We had jobs, paid bills and threw more parties. We must have gone to classes, though I remember very little of that. Still, I made the dean's list every semester.

I met Josh when I was 18 years old. By then, I had already lost my virginity in a garage while taking LSD just before freshman year of high school and spent a few years doing any illegal drug that didn't require a needle. I watched my best friend become fairly addicted to speed, and I found I had the courage to tell her parents (who refused to believe me). Then I quit doing drugs, got a full-time job and, of course, *lived on my own* (according to me at least). I almost never feel like I missed out.

Josh is the love of my life. Early in our relationship, he let me paint his toenails purple. Some people think this is weird, but to me it said, "I'll do anything for you." When he took me home for Christmas that weekend with his toenails still painted, it said "And I want my family to know exactly how I feel." I took the whole thing as a very romantic gesture.

The first time I noticed him, he was working behind the bar at a restaurant where I was waiting tables. There was a computer behind the bar that you could clock in and out from, but there was also one in the dining room. I didn't feel like going over to the dining room so, while talking to a friend, I asked him if he would clock me out. I was used to being able to ask for something with a smile and get what I wanted. He barely looked at me. "I'm busy," he said. "Clock yourself out." I was shocked. And that's when I noticed *he was kind of cute*.

We hung out for six months without kissing. He brought me flowers, took me on picnics and bike rides, and stayed over late into the night talking while he rubbed my legs. Soon after our first kiss, we had our first argument. I told him it didn't seem like it was going to work out. He looked at me like I was crazy. "What are you talking about? Just because we have an argument you think we have to break up? What about working through it?" He shook his head and laughed. Breaking up because of an argument seemed so ludicrous to him that he didn't even take me seriously. His parents have been married for 40 years.

Five years later, he asked me to marry him. We had been living together for four.

I came home from yoga and the house was spotless. Fresh purple irises were on the table and he'd made dinner. Over a bottle of champagne, he told me that his stomach hurt. I knew he was going to propose and somehow it didn't bother me at all that it appeared to be making him sick! I knew he loved me. I knew I wanted to marry him.

It was easy to say yes.

It didn't occur to me then that my first encounter with Josh, when he refused to clock me out, was an indicator of the sometimes subtle and sometimes not-so-subtle battle that would exist between us from that moment forward. We may be living the dream life in Hawaii, we may love each other very much . . . but we have always fought.

I don't know how to do yoga with Josh or in my marriage. I don't know how to inhale and pause, how to exhale and connect more deeply when the going gets tough. It's as if I live a double life between home and the yoga studio, or even home and my practice.

Now he asks, "Why can't you just put things away? Why can't you just finish what you start? Why would you leave the last two dishes in the sink instead of just finishing the fucking job???" He says it when he just can't take it anymore, when he has ignored it for as long as he can and maybe when he's not living up to his own expectations either. "I want to!" I say, "I swear. I want to be organized and respectful and have a happy marriage where my husband isn't disappointed in me. But it's *hard*." Sometimes I pick up my piles with resentment. *Is this the only way I will ever be good enough for him? Pick up the stupid pile of paperwork, put the breakfast dishes in the dishwasher, hurry, get my clothes off the bathroom floor, hurry, before he sees.*

Then he complains about the pile on the dresser. *Whatever. I can't do it. I will never be able to be like his mother who worked full-time and then spent every other waking moment taking care of the housework, the cooking, the bills—everything always taken care of for her children and her husband. Forget it, I'm not interested. It's just not possible for me. This marriage is never going to work.*

But then, later, he pulls me toward him in bed and turns me around so that we fit together. Every question I have about whether or not we should be together disappears. When we sleep, some part of us keeps touching; his hand is on my stomach or my leg is over his back or our ankles are intertwined.

I read once that if you recorded a couple at night and watched how they slept together, you could determine if their relationship would last. Touching while you sleep is a good sign. During the times when I feel the most distant in our relationship, the most concerned that maybe this isn't going to work, I reach over with my hand or my foot in the middle of the night and make contact, hoping that it will help. And it feels in those moments like it might.

When things get hard between Josh and me we actually wonder if having a baby will help. But I really don't know if I want kids. A woman once told me, with tears in her eyes, "It's the first time you will ever know what it's like to truly put something else before yourself. You might not think of yourself as selfish, you might think you put other people before you all the time, you might think this, until the day you birth your first child. Only then will you know that you have never wholly put anyone or anything else before you like this." She was dreamy when she said it, blindly and unconditionally loving in a way that was foreign to me.

I picture her every time I ask the question, every time Josh asks, do I want kids? Her image is not the thing that makes me long to be a mother. It's actually the thing that makes me fear it the most, that makes me want to turn the other direction and run from a future where I will no longer have the freedom to put myself first.

But I'm curious. I love to know what people are

talking about, to understand why they feel or act the way they do. Sometimes when I watch horrible things happen to someone in a movie I wonder... *What would it be like to feel that kind of pain or fear or sadness?* There's a desire to feel it for myself, to understand fully. And so sometimes I say, "Yes, I do want kids, let's do it." Then he says no. Just when I start to think he's right, he changes his mind. But it's always a moment too late. I am already afraid again, sure I don't want kids anymore.

One day we both say yes on the same day, and just like that we start to try. This is how I first learn about ovulation. (I know nothing about it until I read my first book on getting pregnant.) I realize that I had gone to a clinic three different times as a teenager, worried about some sort of STD because no one, including the doctors at the clinic, had ever told me that, "Cervical fluid that resembles 'egg whites' is a sign that you are near ovulation or are ovulating."

We begin to have more sex, a lot more sex, and we fight a lot less. Is it the sex or the excitement of doing something new, of creating a whole new life for ourselves, that lessons the fighting? My mom would say the sex. Josh would say the sex. My mom is always telling me that sex needs to be a priority in my marriage. She says if I'd rather sleep, watch a movie, work, or be alone then my priorities are fucked. "If you're too tired because you worked so long, you might as well get a divorce because if your job is more important than your marriage, your marriage is over." It is a powerful wake-up call. Josh says it relieves his stress and if he's less stressed he won't get so irritated at me. For seven months we have a lot of sex. Not just when I'm ovulating either, because the trying-to-get-pregnant-sex is a reminder that I actually really enjoy having sex with my husband.

And for seven months I pee on sticks. One day I wake up and my boobs hurt. It's a sign I'm going to start my period, and I feel a little bit of relief. I am not even going to bother peeing on another stick only to find myself staring at another pink minus symbol. Suddenly I don't feel so sure I want a baby anymore. I have a good life, with freedom, and opportunity for selfish indulgences. A few days later I still haven't started my period and I have one stick left, still sitting on the bathroom counter. Josh is watching TV in the living room when the plus sign appears in the window.

I inhale and the breath gets stuck inside me. My mouth is open as my back slides down the bathroom wall. Part smiling, part bewildered, part excited and part in total disbelief, I sit on our newly remodeled bathroom floor for at least five minutes before placing the stick on the edge of the bathtub and walking out into the living room.

The words won't come out. I stand staring at him and I just keep repeating myself "Um, I'm, uh, I'm . . ." Finally, "I'm pregnant."

I'm happy. We're both very happy. We only tell our parents and two or three of my friends, since all the books I'm reading advise, "Do not tell people you are pregnant until you've reached the second trimester."

My boobs get big and I get tired. My hands rest frequently on my belly and I treasure any visual sign of growth. I love the physical changes, but the rest is pure misery. I want to sleep and I want to throw up all the time, but I rarely do. I envy the pregnant women who actually do throw up every day because I imagine that they at least feel better afterward, whereas I am miserable all day long. I try keeping crackers by the bed, eating hard-boiled eggs in the middle of the night, toast before getting up, snacking all day long, sucking on lemon candy, drinking fresh ginger tea and sparkling water. I read every "Top Ten Tried and True Tricks for Managing Morning Sickness" article I can find and then I just lay on the floor of the yoga studio and moan.

Since I see yoga as the cure for every ailment on earth, I expect to feel great the entire pregnancy. But instead, the smell of cooking, the thought of eating and the sight of nearly every kind of food makes me want to vomit. I don't quite understand why my yoga practice hasn't spared me of this.

At work, I pretend to be fine, or if it's really bad I say I have food poisoning. I only have to put on a serious show for the few hours a day when I teach classes. The rest of the time I hide behind the curtains and avoid the world.

At home, Josh takes care of me. He cooks all the

food, does the dishes, tells me to rest or go to bed. He rubs my feet, my head and my back. When I'm eleven weeks pregnant, a student asks me if I've gotten a boob job. Although I still have seven days before transitioning into the second trimester, I decide to tell my Saturday morning class of 25 students. "I want to let everyone know . . . I didn't get a boob job."

Thank You

"If the only prayer you ever say in your entire life is thank you, that would suffice."

– Meister Eckhart

August 20th came and went. I had been pacing my neighborhood for weeks, having read that walking may naturally induce labor. A month earlier, I had shown up at the doctor's office in a panic because the birth of a 13-pound monster baby was all over the news, and since I'd had only one ultrasound early on ... *how could we be sure this baby wasn't going to be 13 pounds?*

The doctor wraps the measuring tape around my stomach and back. She says my belly's seemingly massive size is an optical illusion because I am petite. It turns out the measurements show I'm on the small side of average.

Still, in Home Depot, I get a sympathetic look in every aisle. People tell me I'm huge, they say I must be having twins, I have the biggest belly they've ever seen. It confuses me to be seen as large, after a lifetime of trying to gain weight because I thought I was too skinny. It shocks me to learn that people will say such things to a pregnant woman. I vow to never tell a pregnant woman she looks huge.

Many years later, I went to visit my very petite friend who was eight months pregnant with twins. I was driving to visit her in Berkeley while coaching myself in the car...*do NOT say she looks huge, do not say she looks huge.* I thought the optical illusion factor might shock me and I wanted to be ready. I over pre-pared though because when I saw her what came out was, "Oh! You look much smaller than I was expect-ing." She snapped at me that the babies were healthy.

She explained later that she'd been struggling to gain enough weight during the pregnancy and that this had been an ongoing concern. So I revised my philosophy: Never comment on a pregnant woman's size and always tell her she looks absolutely beautiful.

I expect to gain 25 pounds because the pregnancy books I'm reading say the average for my height and pre-pregnancy weight of 110 pounds is between 25 and 35 pounds. Having been thin my whole life, I assume the same will be true during pregnancy.

I'm planning to have a homebirth...in a horse trough filled with water. My doctor has been delivering babies at home for 24 years on the island and, of course, any self-respecting yoga teacher would have a homebirth if possible, *right?*

The scale at my doctor's office is in the bathroom. The doctor asks me to go in, weigh myself, then come out and tell her what it says. I told her the truth at 117 pounds, at 128 pounds, 132 pounds, and 136 pounds. But when I look down and see the line on the scale rest at 142, I suddenly feel ashamed. I go back into her office and with no premeditation whatsoever I hear myself say "138."

I have a picture of myself on my due date in a bathing suit standing by the boat launch at the beach park less than a mile from our house. With the same skinny arms and legs I've always had, I appear to be doing a magic trick in order to stand upright given the size of my 35-pound belly. Although I was sick to death of hearing it and literally thought I might punch the next person to say so . . . they were all right. My belly looked HUGE.

That day Josh and I pile into a 2.5 person kayak along with our dog, our new friend Katie and my giant belly. The waves, the dog and the fact that we are over capacity in the kayak makes us capsize in the middle of the ocean. We flip. I am grateful for all the Chaturangas (yoga push-ups) that make it possible for me to hoist myself back up into the kayak sideways, with no ground to jump from, while quite possibly carrying two 13-pound babies in my giant belly. Josh is impressed. I'm proud. For the first time I want to tell the truth about how much weight I've gained. But I don't.

Katie is going to cover all my classes at the yoga studio for six weeks. I interviewed her over the phone and she came to Hawaii from Southern California. She's staying in the *ohana* (studio apartment attached to our house), and since there's no kitchen back there she uses ours. Tonight, like every other, she's cooking stir-fry with olive oil, cashews, cauliflower, broccoli, and soy sauce. She has irritable bowel syndrome (IBS) and cooks pretty much the same dinner for herself every night. Sometimes she adds shrimp or scallops and sometimes it's zucchini instead of broccoli. She uses one cutting board, meticulously slices each type of vegetable, and re-wraps the unused portion for the following day. Everything fits into one small frying pan, and from there, into one small bowl. The kitchen is clean before dinner is even ready. Then she sits down and eats as slowly and meticulously as she has cooked, chewing every bite completely before readying for the next. Food finally smells good to me.

Five days after my due date, I go into labor, two days later, Kalia is born. I wake up the first night of labor with the sensation of light cramping. I lie awake in my bed willing the contractions to get stronger, but all through the night there is only a mild discomfort every 10 or so minutes. The next day, I can do pretty much anything I want, though every 10 minutes I still have to pause and take a few deep breaths to get through the contractions. I am comforted by the degree of sensation. It isn't so bad. I read to lean in to the sensation rather than to resist, and to breathe. I read that natural childbirth could be pain-free and I have every intention of having a natural, pain-free childbirth. My mom is hurt that I read about my labor instead of seeking advice from her, who also had two children at home.

That evening, the contractions start to get stronger. By midnight, I'm convinced the baby's coming soon, and Josh calls our homebirth doctor, Jacquie. My contractions are much stronger now and I feel more pain in my back than in my belly. As hours of labor pass, I get pissed at the ass who wrote the stupid book I read about pain-free childbirth and pissed at myself because I should have known better since a man wrote it! But for now, I'm just breathing slowly and deeply as much as I can.

After 19 more hours of back labor, I begin to worry. I ask Jacquie if I can go to the hospital. She says no and tells me it's too late for that. We are an hour from the hospital and I need to be comfortable. "You can do this," she says. But she stalls again when I ask her to check how far I've dilated. Every time she's checked for the past 15 hours, nothing has changed. Later I realize she was stalling because she knew I wasn't dilating and didn't want to discourage me with news I didn't want to hear.

Everyone says walking will help, but the pain in my back is so intense I can't stand, let alone walk. Mostly I sit on my living room floor with my head on the coffee table, or I lie in my bed. Someone is always rubbing my back. My mom; Josh (of course); my friend Andrea, who's in nursing school; Jacquie; Jacquie's assistant, who's also an acupuncturist; and Katie comes and goes. Everyone rubs my back.

Finally, it's time to push. I'm in a horse trough filled with warm water. Bob is in the other room now. Katie is here. Josh is hunched over the side of the trough rubbing my back and, for the first time since labor began, I start to cry. *I'm done. I can't do it anymore.* I believe myself completely. I try to give up, as if I have that choice. "I can't do it. I can't do it." I start repeating aloud.

My mom tells me "Just ONE more honey. You can do it, just one more." I can't bear the thought of believing that it's only one more if that isn't true.

I turn to Jacquie. "This is the only one that matters," she says.

I understand this. Let go of everything else that has happened. Don't worry about what may happen next. Just be right here, right now, in this moment. And these words save me. I take a deep breath and push again . . . and again and again because, no, that wasn't the last one. There's a pink and orange striped beach towel folded over one side of the trough and I bite down on the towel covered plastic rim and push. I push as hard as I can. Jacquie tells me to wait, I think she wants to stretch me so I won't tear, but I say no. I can't wait. I have to push. So I do.

The baby comes out with the umbilical cord

wrapped around her neck, but I don't know this until Josh tells me later—it happens so fast. Jacquie spins her around in the water to unwrap the cord and puts her right into my arms. Later I see the photos of me holding a dark blue baby and I cry. Thank you God . . . *thank you, thank you, thank you for letting her be OK.*

As those words rise spontaneously from deep in my heart, I begin to panic. I don't believe in God and yet I am suddenly desperate to believe. For the very first time in my entire life, I feel the need to depend on something bigger than humanity. I need a higher power to pray to, someone to lie down on the ground and plead to. I am supposed to be responsible for this innocent baby girl for the rest of my life, yet I feel helpless. Anything can happen. So much is going to happen that I can't control, that no human being could. I need a higher power on my side, and it occurs to me: I need God's blessing, the blessing I shunned on my wedding day.

Though I don't really understand it, out of desperation, I begin to pray. I pray that she will be safe, that no one will hurt her, that fifth grade girls won't humiliate her and break her heart, that her teenage years won't tear us apart, that I will be a good mother, that she will be safe, that I will know what to do. . .and again and again that she will be safe, and again and again . . . *thank you God.*

Plus One

"It seems to me that the idea of a personal God is an anthropological concept which I cannot take seriously."

— Albert Einstein

I did not want God to be at my wedding. I wasn't even comfortable saying the "G-word." My best childhood friend was raped by her step-father, a self-proclaimed "Man of God" who was active in her community church. For three years, he suffocated her with chloroform and took pictures of her naked body.

When I visited her each summer, he would lead us in prayer after dinner each night. He used the "G-word" a lot.

When I was planning my wedding, I associated God with religious, self-righteous and judgmental hypocrisy. I had a serious chip on my shoulder about random comments and claims that seemed, in my mind, to come from "those people who believe in God." I lumped all of "those people" into a single category of people who believe the entire population of the planet, (with the exception of those who share their exact faith), will spend eternity in Hell. Even if someone lives in a faraway jungle and has simply never heard about God, too bad, they will still be punished with eternal suffering for not being a believer. "They" also preach about being tolerant and loving, saying that God loves all, unless of course you're gay, then "they" believe God may have invented AIDS to punish and kill you.

They might also take pictures of themselves molesting a 16-year-old girl and cut the pages from their bible so they can store the Polaroids there.

What I understood about God then and the people who used that name seemed ridiculously offensive. God—as an ego-driven deity who plays favorites, has temper tantrums, demands restitution, and punishes all those who do not behave as he commands—repulsed me. I didn't like to hear his name, to say his name, to believe that he existed, or to connect with others who believed in him. So why on earth would I invite *him* to my wedding?

On the other hand, when we have to make a choice between getting the approval of someone and honoring our own deepest desire, we sometimes choose the approval. How many brides have never compromised on their guest list anyway?

Lyn is a minister of the psychic church. I didn't really know what that meant on the day we asked her to marry us, but because of my association to the word and the meaning of God, I assumed it meant she would not be speaking about him. She is not religious in the way I understood religion. So when the word first came out of her mouth and I discovered that this was not the case, I asked if I could write the ceremony myself. Not just our vows, but the entire ceremony from beginning to end.

"It would make it feel more personal," I said. I didn't want to offend her. She was my soon-to-be mother-in-law's friend since high school. We first met five years earlier when I attended the baptism of her grandchild. I went with Josh as his date. We were in her living room, and Josh's ex-girlfriend was there, too. I couldn't remember her saying anything about God then.

In any case, if I had to write every word of my wedding ceremony to keep him away, I would.

The day before the wedding, we were sitting in white metal folding chairs outside a vacation rental house on the Big Island of Hawaii. Lyn was holding the manila folder with the script I had written for the ceremony inside. She read it. Everything seemed fine. Lyn was looking directly at me when she said, "I'd like your permission to say a few words before I begin to read from the script." I was smiling, of course. "I think it is important and appropriate that we ask for God's blessing on this occasion."

I was still smiling. It was the most sincere looking smile I could construct, though it was not sincere at all. It was entirely meant to form the persona of someone that Lyn would approve of. My heart beat loudly and I felt hollow inside. I wondered if she could hear it. Disappointment filled my body and squeezed at the base of my neck. I was torn. I didn't want to offend her. I wanted her to like me, and yet, in this moment, I didn't like her at all anymore. I didn't want God's damn blessing. And this was *my* wedding.

I shifted and switched the cross of my legs, laced my fingers together, and a long nervous breath passed through me. I was still smiling when I responded, "I guess that would be fine." She smiled with approval, which I was grateful for. I thought, *maybe no one will notice*. I was oblivious to the possibility that not every one of my friends and family felt the same way I did about God. I completely forgot that my dad is a "Born Again."

Later, as we stand in front of family and friends, I wonder if anyone can see the stiffness in my face and neck when she asks for God's blessing. Despite all of my efforts to keep him away, all of my judgments, discomforts and absolute refusal to send him an invitation, he came anyway—as a "plus one."

Upon his arrival, I endured his presence with indignation, without connection or gratitude. Then, quickly, I forgot about him as I kissed my new husband every time the glasses clinked. The sun set behind us and filled the sky with blazing color and we made new memories with our family and friends, shared wine, listened to the rolling waves of the Pacific Ocean and I never even noticed if God was still around.

Months before our wedding day, I cried as we signed the agreement to get married at this hotel, real tears of sadness, because I thought it was stuffy and staged and snobby. We were planning to get married at a bed-and-breakfast up the hill, but the owner double-booked us with another couple.

That day was September 11th 2001, when we visited the six places that were still available. We saw the news that morning—the images of the Twin Towers collapsing—but we didn't have all the details yet and . . . we had everything scheduled. So even though it felt a little strange, we continued on with our plans.

Of the places we visited, this hotel was the only option remotely acceptable, and it was right on the beach. We sat on a bench with the ocean behind us, near the lawn where the ceremony would take place. We signed the contract, I smiled brightly and thanked the woman who worked at the hotel. We said goodbye, and when she walked away . . . I started to cry. While buildings crumbled and thousands of people were dying in New York City, others screaming, lost, burning, and some even jumping to their deaths for fear of being burned alive–while thousands more were losing people they loved–I sat and cried because I was going to get married at a place that made me feel like a snob. On a beach. In Hawaii. And my soon to be husband comforted me.

Cori Martinez

Practice

I have to put my mat on the floor by my bed or I might not get on it. Even then, I only spend a few minutes on it.

I couldn't care less about handstands.

When I teach, I inhale deeply and exhale completely. I tune in to the movements of the students, the room and the words that flow from my lips.

I love teaching.

For now, my practice is my teaching, but I'm not sure if that counts.

At home, Kalia cries. She barely ever sleeps. She

just keeps crying. Some people say it gets easier. Some people cruelly, I think, say it gets harder. It's hard now.

I hold her and my neck hurts from looking down. I breathe in and out until she finally falls asleep in my arms. I know not to put her down if I want her to stay asleep. I hold her and sit on my yoga mat. I close my eyes, listening, feeling, thankful.

This too is my practice now.

Kalia

"Silence is a source of Great Strength."

– Lao Tzu

The night Kalia is born I have a large stack of organic cotton receiving blankets, organic cotton onesies, organic cotton cloth diapers and an organic cotton bath towel stacked up by the bed. I have a rule that she will only wear organic cotton clothing.

After a 44-hour labor and a water birth in a horse trough, everyone goes home and Josh and I are left with a baby that hasn't stopped screaming since she came out. We can't quite get the diapers on right . . . or the clothes . . . or the blanket . . . and she keeps pooping every couple of hours.

I sprained my back, lost a lot of blood and can't walk or sit upright. I had no idea it would be this hard. She just keeps screaming. And pooping. All night long. By morning, every organic piece of cotton in the house is dirty and our (still nameless) baby is clothed in a regular cotton onesie from Wal-Mart. If I had gotten the message, I may have softened my grip on all that I had decided was required of a good mother. But I wasn't listening.

Kalia is six weeks old when my dad comes to visit.

My dad. Before he came into my room when I was nine and told me he was leaving, he used to push me on the Big Bird swing in our backyard, chase me around the dining room table, and finish my leftovers. He even taught me how to ride a bike. But after he kissed me goodbye that night, he didn't seem to know how to keep being my dad. And I didn't know how to be his daughter. I dated Josh for five years, before he ever even met my dad.

Still, I asked my Dad to walk me down the aisle. As we waited for the song that is our cue to walk, I let tears well up in my eyes and I said, "I don't think I can do this." The moment I heard my own words, I knew they weren't true. But they made me need my dad, made him have to step up and be my father and say the thing, whatever it would be, that would make it OK to walk.

I don't even remember what he said, but since I really had no doubts, anything would have worked, and it did. I saw the beginning of tears in his eyes, too, as he remembered. I imagined him thinking. . . *Oh, this is how it's done.* We walked arm in arm, father and daughter. That was five years ago and I haven't seen him since.

Today, he is coming to meet his first grandchild. He is supposed to be bringing my Grandma, but he arrives with a pink onesie instead. A week earlier, my grandmother had gone to sleep next to her husband of 29 years and didn't wake up. This was the first meaningful death of my life.

My grandma and grandpa (who married when I was one) used to travel the country, or maybe it was only the coast of California, in an RV. They would come stay in our driveway for weeks, and when it was time for them to go, I would stand at my bedroom window and cry. They had filled me with their banjo music and the lyrics to "You Are My Sunshine," with card games, stories, and ham sandwiches on white bread. I longed to run outside and charge through the door of the green and white RV to interrupt their daily game of Scrabble. But they always drove away.

My grandpa will sell the RV now that my grandma is gone for good. I should have called her more often these past few years. I should have mailed her those pictures. She never even saw a picture of her great-grandchild. I am terrible at those things, at keeping in touch.

I park the car in the airport parking lot and walk across the street to the single baggage claim carousel. The moment he sees us, my dad goes straight for Kalia. He has a clean slate with her. I can feel his longing to be her grandfather, can see the hope that he would be . . . *or is he completely oblivious? Does he think all it takes is a bloodline?*

He must have known it took more, because he comes back three times over the next few years. When I move back to California, he comes for her birthdays. After my grandpa dies, he starts to come for Christmas, sometimes for Thanksgiving and Christmas both.

At the airport, as usual, Kalia cries the moment she goes into the car seat. My dad sits in front with me, even though I wish he'd sit in back with her. He tells me she'll be fine. We have the usual 35-minute drive ahead of us to get home from town. I pull over after 10 minutes. Kalia's face is covered with patches of red; she is screaming at the top of her lungs. I am trying to be calm as I explain to my dad that we'll probably have to stop a few times on the way home. He laughs. His confidence that she is OK annoys me. What does he know about newborns? My mom probably did all the work with us. Plus it was so long ago. Kalia is hysterical and soon I will be too.

We pull off the only highway on the island, into a scenic pullout, which is there for the tourists to stop and take pictures of the Pacific Ocean. The speed limit on the one-lane highway is only 55 miles per hour, but without these scenic pullouts the tourists will drive 20 miles per hour to see the breathtaking view that is my daily commute. Since Kalia was born, this commute has become the very worst part of my life. I hate it now as she screams.

I take her out of her car seat and begin to breastfeed. Her eyes are swollen shut and so she blindly searches for my nipple, opening and closing her mouth as her body continues to shake. A few minutes later she's calm, which somehow makes me feel worse, because I know we're not done yet.

She starts screaming as soon as I put her back in the carseat. My dad laughs. I am too insecure to pull over again.

Throughout his first visit with Kalia, my dad wants to hold her a lot. When she starts to cry in his arms, I get up to take her and he turns the other direction. "She's fine," he says. It drives me crazy. I am sure I can make her stop. But that might not be true.

I sit down anxiously and watch them. She keeps

crying, and he keeps walking and patting her back. He's not anxious, nervous or uncomfortable. He's not blaming himself or feeling like a failure. He's not desperate for her to stop, tortured by the sound of her screams. He just walks and pats her on the back. He hums, and his hums don't sound increasingly frantic like mine sometimes do. He holds her till she falls asleep and then he sits down in the rocking chair and falls asleep with her in his arms. It seems to me like he's been a father before.

Maybe more of one than I'd ever noticed. By the time my dad leaves, I have a new perspective to consider. *Maybe he never forgot how to be a dad. Maybe I just stopped letting him.*

Months pass and still, no matter what I do, Kalia just keeps screaming. I have changed my diet, cut out acidic foods, gassy vegetables, then strong flavors, then dairy, and then when I am eating only rice and eggs, I read that maybe I should cut out eggs. I swaddle her, shush her, sing to her, bounce her, rock her, and still she cries.

Because she'll wake up crying if I lay her down,

I hold her while she sleeps for nearly the first nine months of her life. Tired and sometimes defeated, other times overwhelmed by my love, I close my eyes and listen to the sound of her tiny breath. It is quiet and, often as I sit, I feel the depth and clarity of this quiet. This is how I first discover a practice that has nothing to do with yoga postures or rules of behavior, a practice of listening and discovering space and peace.

For six years, I've been doing the physical practice of yoga, stretching and strengthening my body while deepening and lengthening my breath. I have discovered subtleties in the physical postures, small minute shifts and inner actions that wash away the outer tensions of my inner struggles and leave me with a sense of ease. But I've truly never sat in meditation until now.

Holding my finally sleeping baby, without a single Downward Dog, in the quiet of my own mind is where I meet God as I have never imagined. It is a place where the voice of shame, doubt, regret, and the emotions of anger, sadness, and guilt don't need to be resisted, but can instead be allowed and held with love, a place where it is very, very, quiet and yet infinitely vast and profound.

Here, I am at peace.

Cori Martinez

Ahui Ho

(Hawaiian for "Until We Meet Again")

"He nods, as if to acknowledge that endings are almost always a little sad, even when there is something to look forward to on the other side."

— Emily Giffin,
Love the One You're With

Many people move to Hawaii with dreams of a life in paradise. Then, three months later, having discovered that—in paradise—there are cockroaches, limited jobs, and no home garbage pickup, they pack their bags to return to the mainland.

No one is ever in a hurry, even when they're an hour late. "Hawaiian time" means you better get used to waiting.

It costs thousands of dollars for a family to leave Hawaii, so vacations off the island are expensive, though less than a few months worth of groceries, considering it costs about a hundred dollars to leave the grocery store with one bag of food.

It rains hard and heavy and a lot.

Not all restaurants have bathrooms, and none of the bathroom sinks have hot water.

Although there are eight Thai and four sushi restaurants, there's no Indian, Chinese, Mexican, or Italian food. There's only one coffee shop and it doesn't have Wi-Fi or an espresso maker.

There's one gym and it doesn't have a sauna or a steam room, unless you count the fact that the locker room is so damp with humidity and bodily fluids that the plug-in fan on the counter blowing wet smelly air at you actually feels good.

Sometimes all this is just more than an eager newcomer can bear. When someone moves to Hawaii from the mainland and stays less than a year, it's said that the island simply refused to "embrace" them.

On the other hand, those who are lovingly embraced by the island accept the cockroaches, find a job or start a new business, and buy a pickup truck so they can take their own garbage to the "transfer station."

We buy a pickup truck. We also tent the house to kill the termites and get milk from the gas station or fresh from the cow on the Amish farm (depending on the time of day when we suddenly need it since the grocery store is 30 miles away). We walk in the rain, swim in the rain, and quit talking because we can't hear each other anymore over the sound of the rain pounding down on the metal roof of our house. We pay $6 for hummus, $9 for orange juice, and vacation on the other side of the island. We are embraced for seven years and think we'll stay forever.

Then one day, we decide to go. We want options for Kalia that aren't available here. We miss the mainland, the abundance of diverse foods and cultures. We miss traveling and we miss certain friends.

Although it feels like a very right decision, it is far from easy.

My mom begins sobbing when we tell her. I think Bob is angry. It breaks my heart. We came here to build a multi-million dollar mushroom farm as a family. Though we have built the farm, it's seven years later and we still aren't done. My mom and Josh hold the leading roles in the company, and they often don't get along, leaving Bob and I often equally in the middle. Sometimes, we are brilliant moderators. Other times, Bob has consumed an entire bottle of single malt Scotch by midday and I am emotional and resentful of everyone.

I just want to live a peaceful, happy life. I want everyone to love each other and get along. Instead, my mom is crying again and Josh is yelling again and Bob is drunk again and I want everyone to be different than they are again, and none of us remembers yesterday when we all had a beautiful picnic at the beach.

We've had so many beautiful days at the beach.

I moved here as a recent college graduate, in

love and lust for a future in paradise. I got married, became an entrepreneur, a homeowner, a teacher and a member of a community. I found friendships, support and courage. I struggled through a humbling transformation into motherhood and smile almost daily into the eyes of my beautiful, almost two-year-old baby girl as we hold hands in the shallow pool of the ocean.

I opened my body, my mind, my heart, and learned to breathe in the wind on my skin, to sense the graceful ebb and flow of the ocean that surrounds me deep within my own body and life.

My yoga studio is a booming success.

Though I'm smiling, tears stream down my face when I, once again, open up to my Saturday morning class: "I am moving back to the mainland."

Cori Martinez

Practice

The room is hot again. This time ninety degrees. I move with my breath, slower than anyone else in the room, but still faster than I've moved in a long time.

Inhale, Up Dog. Exhale, Down Dog. Inhale, Warrior One. Exhale, Warrior Two. Inhale, Reverse Warrior Two. Exhale, Vinyasa. Then the left side. Right side again. Left side again. Then a hundred thousand more times on each side, then some core work on fast forward, then some arm balances. Everyone else keeps going, even if they're fumbling. I laugh, thinking *maybe it's a joke. Seriously? We're still going?* I take Child's Pose.

Cori Martinez

Class is fun. the music is loud. Anne Marie makes me laugh. but I don't quite fit with Hot Power Yoga. I practice here. I teach here. My class is called Slow-Flow. At first, I wouldn't wear the cordless mic. but then I do and honestly... I do feel pretty cool. I think that's partly why we use it.

I talk a lot. I'm trying to convince everyone around me to slow down. without actually saying so, except I actually cue students to slow down. I want the students to like Slow-Flow Yoga, but mostly they don't. Of course some do. I want desperately for everyone to see their whole lives as yoga and I try too hard.

I talk about Hawaii like I'm name-dropping, "My studio... in Hawaii." I can't bring myself to sell Yoga Centered when we leave. I don't even try because I am just not ready. I'm convinced we might move back. For now, I fly back every other month with Kalia.

In Sacramento. I eat pork belly. I drink wine, like I used to before yoga.

Exhale, Down Dog. Inhale. right leg up. Exhale, knee to elbow. Inhale. right leg back up. Exhale. knee to elbow. Again. Again. Again. Switch sides.

Plus One... Finding God on the Yoga Mat

Finally Savasana. I lie down on my mat, damp from head to toe, though there's no puddle of sweat around me like there is for some people. The music gets even louder. Eventually, it stops and there is quiet for just a brief moment before it's time to move my fingers and toes, roll to my right side, and come up to sitting. I chant Om. Just once. Like I have to, because everyone else is.

Something in me settles and I feel the ocean I've been missing in the vibration of Om... Until the room erupts with applause.

For the teacher? For the practice? For themselves? I'm not sure, but in any case, I find it odd. Yet I love that everyone around me is smiling.

Cori Martinez

Teaching Power Yoga

"At the center of your being you have the answer; you know who you are and you know what you want."

– Lao Tzu

I thought about opening up my own studio since there wasn't much yoga in Sacramento at the time. I found a building I loved in Midtown and even started negotiating the build-out terms and rent. When I found out just before moving that a Vinyasa studio was opening only a few blocks from where I was looking, I thought I missed my chance. I also wondered if maybe I had gained my chance to teach, without the responsibility of owning a studio. *That might be nice.*

I begin teaching at a new studio owned by someone else in a new town where Power Yoga seems to be the most popular style. I understand my pace is slower and my intention with yoga has become more spiritual than it once was, but I still teach a strong practice and I think I can make a place for myself in this new community.

We call my class *Slow Flow* and the Power Yoga classes have twice as many students in them. I teach Slow Flow for a while. Then, because I'm secretly tormented by having the smallest classes, because I've begun to consider that the students in front of me don't want to practice the way I do and it's my responsibility as a teacher to meet them where they are, and because the only place for me to practice is here and I've been having fun, I decide to give teaching Power Yoga a chance.

I loosen up on alignment details, forget about

addressing patterns of unhealthy movement in exchange for the fun of freedom to flow and move. I turn the music up louder and teach at a faster pace. I teach poses and transitions that half the room isn't really ready for. I watch the students push too hard and try anyways as they mimic the pose enough to convince themselves they've got it. Actually, I stop *really* teaching and start just talking, calling out poses. My assists become generic because there's no time for anything more at this pace.

My classes grow a little. I have fun for a while. I convince myself I've expanded my horizons and feel a passion for what I'm teaching...for a while. Eventually, I feel like I'm not doing or teaching yoga anymore.

I tell Anne Marie I'm going to open my own studio. Up the street. I ask her if I can continue to teach at Zuda until I am further in the process. I promise that I won't talk about it with students and that I'll go quietly when the time comes. She graciously says OK. I can't believe I am practically Heather, that first teacher I hired at Yoga Centered. Except that *I will not* promote my new studio while I'm still teaching here.

No Heartbeat

"Though he's barely the size of a kumquat—a little over an inch or so long, crown to bottom—and weighs less than a quarter of an ounce, your baby has now completed the most critical portion of his development. This is the beginning of the so-called fetal period, a time when the tissues and organs in his body rapidly grow and mature.

He's swallowing fluid and kicking up a storm. Vital organs—including his kidneys, intestines, brain, and liver (now making red blood cells in place of the disappearing yolk sac)—are in *place and starting to function, though they'll continue to develop throughout your pregnancy. If you could take a peek inside your womb, you'd spot minute details, like tiny nails forming on fingers and toes (no more webbing) and peach-fuzz hair beginning to grow on tender skin.*

Your baby's limbs can bend now. His hands are flexed at the wrist and meet over his heart, and his feet may be long enough to meet in front of his body. The outline of his spine is clearly visible through translucent skin, and spinal nerves are beginning to stretch out from his spinal cord. Your baby's forehead temporarily bulges with his developing brain and sits very high on his head, which measures half the length of his body. From crown to rump, he's about 1 1/4 inches long. In the coming weeks, your baby will again double in size—to nearly 3 inches."

I am 10 weeks pregnant, reading about the baby's current development on babycenter.com.

Nine months ago we decided we wanted another baby. It took seven months of dedicated effort. We obviously began to have more sex. It was just like the movies. "OK, it's time. You have to come home right now. I only have 30 minutes! Hurry up!!!"

When the pink plus sign shows through the window this time, I call Josh right away and tell him over the phone. This time we tell *everyone* right away. Family, friends, people at work. I tell all my students. We tell Kalia and she says it's a boy. She is sure of it. She tells everyone about her new baby brother before we ever even have the ultrasound. She tells strangers in the grocery store.

My boobs are big again. I am tired again. I want to sleep all the time and I want to throw up all the time, but I rarely do . . . again.

At ten and a half weeks, I started spotting.

I call the advice nurse at Kaiser and she is very reassuring. Apparently, this happens all the time. Some women spot throughout their entire pregnancy. She asks me all the required questions, which I can tell are required because she seems to be reading them. She concludes that everything is fine and she confirms my appointment for the following week. She says to call back if anything changes or if the bleeding gets worse.

The next morning the bleeding is not worse. Nothing changes. Except I wake up crying, so I call Kaiser again and this time I lie.

I say the bleeding is worse. They give me an appointment for two hours later. I take Kalia to preschool and call Josh. He asks if I want him to meet me there and I say yes, even though it feels a little silly. I'm torn between gut-wrenching fear and feeling the more likely probability that everything is fine. He meets me in the waiting room and comes into the doctor's office with me.

The doctor walks in wearing thick, dark glasses, a light-blue button-up shirt, and khaki pants under his white coat. He smiles. He speaks slowly, moves slowly, taking his time to say hello and check in.

Once my feet are in the stirrups, he asks if I have been bleeding more than this. I smile sheepishly, caught.

"Well, not exactly, I guess I may have overreacted."

Apparently everything looks fine, still intact.

This is a normal amount of spotting, and there is very likely nothing to worry about.

"As long as you're already here though, we can do an ultrasound just to reassure you."

Josh takes my hand. Our one and only ultrasound when I was pregnant with Kalia was a disaster. The technician was either in such a rush or so against our decision to have a naturopathic doctor deliver the baby at home that he spent less than three minutes giving the ultrasound. Two minutes and fifty four seconds to be exact, we recorded the whole thing. Then he said he didn't have time to make a determination about the gender. I cried afterward and wrote him a letter. I told him that he appeared to have forgotten the opportunity he had to be part of some of the most special and memorable moments of people's lives: the first time they hear their baby's heartbeat, and see the shape of its tiny little arms and legs. I told him he had stolen that from me.

This doctor continues to take his time.

He rolls the computer screen closer to me so Josh and I can see it well. I look at Josh and back at the monitor, full of love for this moment. There he is, Kalia's brother, our baby. The doctor traces his arms and legs and head with the pointer until we can fully make out the contours of his little body swimming in the grey and white field. I touch my belly, wanting to reach out and stroke this tiny being that's inside of me.

The doctor has been talking, telling us about what we're seeing, what he's seeing. Then he stops. He quietly asks his assistant to turn down the lights so he can get a closer look at something. He examines the screen closely for a moment and then he looks right into my eyes. I look away from the baby too when he stops talking, and I'm looking at the doctor already before he speaks.

"I'm sorry." He says. "There's no heartbeat."

I hear the words but the translation in my mind and body of what they mean doesn't come right away. It happens in slow motion. *There's no heartbeat.*

I can feel the process of my body sinking and some unknown force rising up from my chest, into my throat and gradually changing the expression on my face. My lips part and I can feel the tightness in my neck and throat that comes when you are just about to cry . . . but I'm waiting. *Maybe he's made a mistake.* I'm waiting for him to tell me he's made a mistake.

"I'm so sorry." He has to repeat. The sound of his voice and the look in his eyes are a promise to me. This is not a mistake. *Oh my God.*

The tears come. And the words continue to echo in my head over and over again. *No heartbeat. No heartbeat. No heartbeat.* I hear myself crying, sobbing and although the pain feels real and the breaking of my heart feels physical, I still somehow doubt this is actually happening.

The doctor hands me a Kleenex and says that he'll give us a few minutes alone. Josh is sitting on the exam table with me now, his arms wrapped around me. Neither of us says or does anything else, other than cry. For me it's the kind of cry where your whole body participates, hands covering a contorted face, eyes squeezed shut, shoulders slumped and shaking. My sobbing stops only long enough for me to gasp for air. Josh has tears, but he isn't crying like that. The

131

doctor comes back at some point.

We have some options. I can have a D&C to remove the fetus from my uterus, I can take pills to induce a miscarriage or I can just wait. I don't know how to decide. When he asks if I know what I want to do I look for an answer, but there's nothing but emptiness. No information comes. I'm in shock. The doctor is apparently going to hand me some more Kleenex, but instead he says, "Oh, my God, I'm out of tissue. I feel like such a jerk. This is the worst day."

For a moment I feel sorry for him. He looks so sad. I wonder what other news he's delivered today. Or was it just this? I'm surprised by his lack of distance from the situation.

"It's OK." I say. But then I start crying again. That is actually the absolute LAST thing I want to hear, even if it's meant for someone else. I don't want anyone to tell me it's OK or that it ever will be. *It's not OK. It's not.* The next thing I absolutely do not want to hear is:

"Don't worry, you can always try again."

Thankfully, this doctor knows enough not to say

that, but many other people over the course of the next few months do not.

I send Anne Marie, the owner of the yoga studio I'm teaching at, a text message:

"Please cover my classes. There's no heartbeat."

Almost two years after I send that message to Anne Marie, I get a text from her: "The baby didn't make it." Now, along with many differences, we have this loss in common.

Obviously we aren't alone. Women have miscarried babies for as long as they have been getting pregnant. I just didn't know about it until I had miscarried my own. People begin to share their stories, which are apparently reserved for the inside crowd. I hear them over and over again for weeks. This is why you're not supposed to tell anyone you're pregnant until the second trimester. The chances of losing the baby during the first three months are greater than any newly pregnant woman wants to face.

Except, then what? You lie around miserable for who knows how long, crying and it's a big mystery why? I didn't mind that people knew. I didn't even mind that much when I would see someone I hadn't talked to in a long time and they would ask me how the new baby was, or how I was handling two kids, or something else like that. Except for Kalia. I wish I had never told Kalia.

The doctor says we can wait to make a decision about what to do. Josh leaves his car at the hospital and drives me home. I crawl into bed. Kalia stays with my mother-in-law, happy as can be to spend extra time with Grandma, oblivious she no longer has a brother. From my bed I send a bulk text to most of the friends in my phone. "The baby has no heartbeat. Please don't call, I'm not ready to talk." All I want to do is cry.

I keep picturing the baby and the future that no longer exists: the birth, the clothes, the relationship between him and Kalia. The doctor never actually says the baby was a boy, but I had taken to referring to it this way based on Kalia's determination. And my own instinct, maybe. I cry over lost soccer games, lost sleepless nights rocking and nursing, lost family vacations with two kids fighting in the backseat. I cry over a whole lifetime . . . lost, because that's how it seems to me in this moment.

I think about the feeling I have when something horrible happens to someone in a movie, and how even though I know I don't ever want it to happen to me, I become deeply curious what it would be like to feel that kind of pain or fear or sadness.

I'm thinking about that when I make the decision to wait. This is a painful situation I would never wish upon myself, or anyone, and I am drawn toward experiencing it fully. I notice I don't want it to go away quickly; I don't want it to be over. I want to cry and I want to imagine the lost future with this baby, even though it only brings me more pain. Waiting seems to be the thing that will most allow that. So I wait. And I cry day after day in my bed.

A week after seeing the doctor I wake up with something like a memory from during the night. It's as if I'd had a long conversation with the baby. I don't remember the conversation, but I have a new understanding as a result of it.

I realize that this was always the way it was going to be. *Never a toddler. Never a teen. Always only this.* And when we both got exactly what we needed to give and receive from the other, we were going to go our separate ways. I have this sense of having communicated at the highest, most spiritual level, and I calmly trust the message irrefutably to be real and true. It brings me a serenity I'm not sure I've ever felt before as I find myself possessing a deep trust in the unfolding of life.

It is the day before Halloween. I get out of bed and leave the house for the first time to take Kalia to get a costume. She's going to be a princess this year, same as last year, and the year before.

When I pull up to the costume shop, blood begins to pour out from between my legs. For nearly a week I have been lying in bed crying and there was never more than very minimal spotting. This is a massive amount of blood. What if I didn't go to the doctor that day and I wasn't expecting this to happen? I feel relief, grateful to be prepared. I tell Kalia calmly,

"Honey, we can't go get your costume. I'm sick and I need Daddy's help. We have to go home right now, I'm sorry." Her response is truly miraculous.

"OK Mommy."

I drive home and call Josh from the car. He comes out and gets Kalia. I make it into the bathroom, where I remain for a couple of hours. I didn't know it would take so long.

And I didn't know there would be so much blood.

It's especially messy because I have this aversion to flushing the fetus down the toilet. So I hold my hands in the stream of blood that continues to pour out of me. Whenever a large clot comes out I examine it. I don't know if it's my imagination or not when I believe I'm holding the baby in my hands. I put it into a box I prepared in advance. I wonder if I'm crazy. *Is this what crazy people do?* But I can't imagine just flushing it.

Eventually, the bleeding slows enough for me to put a pad on and some new clothes. I wash my pants and underwear under the water in the bathtub, which runs red for several minutes. I clean the blood from the bathroom floor and counter and sink. I have to rinse the washcloth several times. Josh comes to the door and asks me if I'm OK. I mean it when I say yes, although the cramping is intense and also unexpected. When I come out I go right to bed.

I wake up for Kalia's bedtime. I crawl into her bed with her and Josh. She begins to talk about her brother. She has big plans for him. She's going to teach him how to carve pumpkins. She still doesn't know.

"Kalia. I have to tell you something, honey." I pull her into my arms. Josh takes one of my hands.

"Your brother isn't going to be born." She looks at me, confused.

"What do you mean?"

I remember how I didn't comprehend this news from the doctor when he said it to me the first time either. And I remember the moment of understanding. My heart breaks a little more as I wait for this moment to come for her.

"He wasn't strong enough to be born, so he left my body." I say.

Tears well up in her eyes and begin to spill over. She begins to sob in such a familiar way.

"But I want him to be born, Mommy! I want to

hold him!" She lies next to me and cries. I am silent. There's nothing more to say. I watch her and am overwhelmed by an intense love for her.

I feel something else too. I miscarried a baby today and now I'm holding my husband's hand and our daughter as they experience this loss with me . . . and somehow I'm at peace with it.

I can feel the quiet I've found in meditation. I can feel God as I've met him in the silence of my mind, comforting us all in our own silence. Though Kalia cries for a while longer and has more questions later, this night she doesn't ask them. Josh runs his fingers through her hair. I know she will be fine. We all will be. Knowing the presence of God, it feels like everything is going to be fine, forever, like everything can be trusted.

I soften into an unarguable trust in life, and whatever it may bring. I feel right now that it is my own willingness to see God in everything that makes everything sacred and holy.

Everything. Even this.

Cori Martinez

Medicine After
the Miscarriage

"And I found that I can do it if I choose to—I can
stay awake and let the sorrows of the world tear
me apart and then allow the joys to put me back
together different from before but whole once again."
— Oriah Mountain Dreamer,
The Invitation

After the miscarriage, my heart begins to heal although my body continues to bleed. It goes on for weeks. The doctor finally says we've waited as long as we can. I need to have a D&C to surgically remove any leftover, physical traces of the baby from my body. Not doing so could lead to a serious infection. This time I tell Josh I'm fine to go alone.

I undress by the hospital bed and pile my clothes in the chair. It's so cold. The doctor comes in to check on me. How am I doing? OK. Am I ready? Yes. I move onto a rolling bed, and someone begins to push me out of the room and down a hallway. The doctor walks next to me. I don't expect the tears that come. First silently pouring out, and then uncontrollably sobbing. They push me into a walk-in freezer with white walls and giant florescent lights. It is so fucking cold.

When I'm calm again the doctor asks me to bend my knees and open my legs. Then he asks me if I'm a runner. Weird. I hate running. Why is he asking? Because my legs are so lean and yet so strong and defined, he says. What? I want to tell him it's the yoga. I love when yoga gets that reputation. I love that yoga is all I've ever done for exercise, and yes, my body is defined. He comes over and holds my hand.

He says something. I don't know what it is. But

when he says it something clicks and I think . . . *Oh, he's gay.*

He looks at me with such kindness and compassion in his eyes. I start to cry again and then I'm back in the other room, in the other bed, with extra blankets covering me.

What happened? It was over.

"We gave you something to forget."

You did what? Was I unconscious? I didn't know I was going to be under.

"No, you weren't unconscious."

How did I get back in this bed?

"You got back in yourself. After the surgery."

No. I didn't. I couldn't have. I don't remember any of that. I don't remember the surgery. I don't remember coming back into this room and getting these blankets.

"You were completely conscious, we just gave you something to forget."

All this time, what's gotten me through was the opportunity to fully experience this thing. To feel the pain and loss and deep, overwhelming sadness, to know that I could feel those things and still make peace with life was so often what made it all OK. And now they have given me something to forget?

There are more blankets piled on top of me, and a nurse was asking . . . "Are you still cold?" *Still cold? Um, no, I don't think so.*

"You've been really cold. You keep asking for more blankets."

What? I have? Was I sleeping?

"No, it's just the medicine."

Oh yeah, the medicine . . . still helping me to forget.

Another nurse comes in. She tells me her name. She says she knows me from yoga, that she sometimes takes my class. She says she is so sorry and that if I need anything to please let her know.

There are more tears, shaking, sobbing. After she's gone I wonder if she knows this wasn't my choice. Does she know why I had the surgery? I want her to know it wasn't my choice. I didn't have an abortion.

A moment later, I can't remember her name, or what she looked like, or if she had said anything else, or if I had. I ask another nurse. There's a nurse here who does yoga, she was here a few minutes ago, what is her name? She tells me and I repeat it over and over and over again in my mind. But when I get home it's gone. I find a note in my purse, in my own writing and it says, remember the nurse who has taken my class. It's only then that I remember the details I can. I look for her for a while. Who is she? But so far I have never found out. Maybe she was in my class today.

I'm angry at first about the "medicine." But soon it becomes part of the experience. An example of what we do, what I do, and will continue to do if not doing it doesn't become more important to me than anything else in the world.

I think we all want the full human experience, the range of emotions and challenges and joys that we came to this human body to feel . . . but we run from them, afraid, and left empty of what we are here to get. Then, as the deepest part of us efforts to be present in our own lives, there begins a craving, and still too afraid, we watch others on TV instead, and we become addicted to it. An addiction that can so easily be overcome just by realizing we have within us more entertainment and deep raw beauty and captivating, thrilling suspense and drama and discovery and insight, right here within our own experiences, than we will ever find watching the experiences of others.

If we keep checking out of our own lives, we will never be satisfied. Something will always be missing. I might not have wanted to checkout during the experience of losing my baby, but I have certainly chosen to do so on a regular basis in other situations.

The medicine after the miscarriage becomes a reminder for me of how desperately I want to experience my life.

If I experience my life more fully because of losing a baby, if I navigate through each day with an unarguable trust, hand in hand with the wisdom of the universe and my new friend who I can unashamedly call God, then I can trust in my miscarriage and in the medicine that helped me to forget. Remembering the dream I had that the baby and I were meant to give each other only exactly what we both needed, I feel so thankful for what I received.

Practice

Inside it is quiet, even though I can hear the occasional car that drives by on the street outside my suburban house window. I can hear them in front of me, and also from the left and the right. The leaking shower faucet drips, drips, drips, streams for one, two, three seconds and then goes back to dripping. The hot water heater, the house heater, and the laptop computer all hum. The dryer ticks, even though it's not on. A motorcycle drives by. Another car. The walls moan as they settle and shift and settle again. A dog is barking far away. A bird chirps right near the backyard window. There's the whisper of my exhale.

I go inside myself and hear my own thoughts. Planning, working, dreaming. Doubt creeps in . . . there's too much to do, I could never do that, someone else could do it better. I still have so much to learn first. There's too much to learn. I should be a better mom. I should clean the house and be a better wife. I should have more sex with Josh. I shouldn't have left that half eaten apple on the counter. Why am I always so cold? I should turn the heat up. I shouldn't turn the heat up; it's already at 70 and that's just ridiculous. Think about the environment, think about the money, but I'm so cold. I'm such a wimp. My feet are cold, and I have socks and boots on. I shouldn't have my shoes on in the house. I don't like to wear shoes in the house. But I'm cold.

I go inside a little further and I notice. There's some space where it's quiet. It's the space where all the noise seems to rise up from, every inner voice and every outer sound. Before it becomes the sound or the voice, it's part of the silence. I can rest in here and be part of that silence too; I can stay as long as I want. I could stay forever, but I know that soon I will forget that I am this silence, and I will rise up out of it with a loud important voice that needs something. wants something. and I will become the voice instead of the silence. At least that's what I'll believe.

For now. I swim in the silence. I stop and float. I look around and listen to the world from here. The voices are still there; the world is still turning. I can even get up and do the dishes ... or not. I could call someone: I could do anything and keep resting in this silence. It isn't a place to retreat to: it's a place to connect more deeply to everything. to everyone. It feels like the only thing that's truly real.

This is what I now call God. This silence that is in me. that is more powerful and real than anything else in my world. This space where anything could happen and it would be OK. more than OK. it would be right.

Cori Martinez

Teacher in Training

"The miracle of love comes to you in the presence of the un-interpreted moment."

– Byron Katie

It's sweet to be teaching again. The students all know about my miscarriage and I don't feel like they expect anything from me when they show up to practice. I don't have it in me just yet to "meet them where they are" in their desire for a Power Yoga practice, and in my eyes they seem finally not to be asking. They seem to simply be supportive and open to whatever I'm able to give right now.

I look around and wonder for the first time if they were ever asking for anything else, or if it was always only me. So concerned with wanting to be liked and accepted, with wanting to have more students in my class . . . Was I the one asking myself to be something I thought they'd want? Plus, wasn't I asking them to be what I wanted them to be? Thinking I was a more evolved practitioner because I moved slower and cared about the details, believing my way was better. Now, I am both humbled by my loss and freed by my discovery of God and my trust in life. Now, I'm not asking them to be anything they're not, I'm not asking that of myself and so I don't feel them asking that of me.

A few weeks later, I tell one student about my plan to open a studio. He's a regular in my class and I'm pretty sure he doesn't go to any other classes here. It seems fair and appropriate for me to tell only him, even given my promise to Anne Marie. But then a few days later I tell three ladies who also come regularly to my class. This gets back to Anne Marie in less than

24 hours and she calls me to say I can't teach there anymore.

She never mentions that I broke my word, but I know she knows. I tell her I understand, and I do. Completely. I ask her then for more than I deserve. Will she please let me teach one final class to say goodbye?

Despite the fact that I truly believed being a studio owner would make me the easiest teacher ever to employ, I was wrong. I have pretty much been an arrogant, high-maintenance teacher since day one. I've barely shown up to meetings, I'm hardly open to feedback, my availability has been extremely limited, I don't like to sub and I've left every other month to fly back to Hawaii, all while my class numbers remain small in comparison to the other teachers.

Now I am planning to open a studio up the street and I've shared this with students at her studio after saying I wouldn't. For some reason, she agrees to let me teach again, even though I can tell she absolutely doesn't want to. Anne Marie has given me everything I've ever asked for since she hired me. I know I've been helpful to her, but I have also been a total pain in the ass. She forgives me though, and we remain friends to this day.

I open Asha Yoga with the help of a new friend who becomes my short-term business partner. The building-out process is once again insanely busy, but soon enough, we're done.

The studio walls are a deep burnt-orange. The grass-cloth sconces dimly light the space. I teach in front of a single, creamy, Venetian-plaster wall that spans the front of the room; its focal point is a reclaimed redwood altar adorned with the Buddha, candles, flowers, and beads. It is possibly the most beautiful yoga studio I have ever seen.

Now that bodies are beginning to regularly fill the space, moving, breathing, and sitting quietly in meditation, it is becoming sacred, safe, and, as so many have commented, womb-like. I love to roll out my mat here, to teach here, to be here. I practice and teach slowly. The room temperature is ambient. I'm not wearing a cordless mic and my classes are filling up.

Of course, I still don't think it's appropriate for me to lead a Teacher Training. Not yet, anyway. I need to know so much more first and I need to be teaching for so much longer. Ten years is nothing.

But then I see teachers around me starting to teach teachers, and they've only been practicing for four or five years, some maybe teaching for three. It makes me eye-rolling annoyed and a little bit shocked. Who do they think they are? I realize that's the same question that keeps me from doing it. Who do I think I am?

It's the same question that keeps me from doing a lot actually. Who do I think I am to take a stand? To share how such an ancient practice can apply to our modern lives? To say something I haven't read in a book or been taught by a master? To write an article of my own? To share from my own experience and evolving beliefs?

My business partner tells me I can teach. She's my ego's cheerleader and she's very convincing. Over the course of four months, I plan a 200-hour Yoga Teacher Training Program, get it registered through

Yoga Alliance, print some flyers, add the info to the website and people begin to sign up.

The next 200 hours make the top ten list of worst experiences of my life. I forget completely about God and trusting in life. Day one: my ego turns on me and gets stuck on repeat, asking, "Who do you think you are?" Over and over and over again. Two members of the group are schoolteachers. One of them looks at me in complete disappointment constantly, and the other offers me suggestions at the end of every session. "You should get a flip chart, or a white board," he says.

The last five days of the training are at a retreat center. I've taught many retreats at a beautiful center in the mountains of Hawaii, overlooking the ocean from a shiny wooden platform with shoji screen walls, eating organic meals, and swimming under a waterfall during the breaks. Everyone was always happy.

This is not that. I made the mistake of choosing the retreat center based on the website photos alone. The sleeping arrangements, the flea infested carpet in our practice area and continuously close quarters with people you didn't choose as friends or roommates, along with the intensity of the schedule, the fear of not understanding the material, of not knowing enough or being enough, and whatever else is going on for each person, begins to eat through the composure of almost every participant.

Some cry. Some yell. One of the schoolteachers drops out. He says it's his back, but I am convinced that if I were doing a better job he'd stay. The other schoolteacher doesn't even look at me anymore. Even if she tried, she might find that I am avoiding her eyes as well. It is all more than I am prepared for, more than I am qualified for and more reasons to keep asking: Who do I think I am?

Throughout the training, I spend many hours with my friend who is a therapist. She coaches me on supporting the emotional dynamics of the group. She coaches me through my own emotional breakdown as well, and I swear to her over and over that, "I will never do this again."

On the final day of training, we sit in a circle and I cry as I speak to the group. But my tears are tears of love. I look around and see how each person in the circle has grown; I can see the work it took them to go through varying degrees of transformation, self-discovery, and study.

As I speak, I begin to recognize my own transformation and growth. In comparison to every Teacher Training I will ever lead in the future, this one was absolutely terrible. But, this is how I learned what it was going to take. With hindsight, I am reminded to trust.

I don't just need to know about yoga . . . I need to know how to hold a group of people steady through thick and thin, how to help them bond with each other so they will be there for each other, how to open their eyes to their own capabilities and their own inner wisdom. I need to know the different ways people learn, the ways we hold ourselves back, the things we are universally afraid of, and how to cultivate both trust and courage.

Yet before I can do any of these things for any group, I need to be able to hold steady within myself, open my own eyes to my own capabilities and inner wisdom, see how I am holding myself back, and feel safe enough and courageous enough to move forward. These last 200 hours deeply inspire me to grow.

I start planning my next Teacher Training days after the first one ends. This time, I take a full twelve months to prepare. I begin a six-month-long training for facilitating intense self-inquiry and I begin an intense self-inquiry practice myself. I read book after book about styles of learning and teaching methodology. I write a 190-page training manual which includes everything that was missing from every Yoga Teacher Training I've ever attended. I write lesson plans, an agenda, and an alternate agenda. Obviously, I get a white board.

On my Self-Inquiry Retreat, my teacher says,

"Take a walk. Look around you. When your eyes rest on something, give it a name; a first generation name such as flower, paper, bug, without adding your story of... beautiful flower, paper that should be in a garbage can, or sweet little ladybug. Remember, this is a silent exercise."

Walking, Day One: *Garbage*. I feel sad. *Why do people just throw their garbage on the ground? People are so inconsiderate. Graffiti.* I imagine gang members and kids without responsible, educated parents. *Can I find beauty in garbage and graffiti? Tree. I wish there were more trees. This would be easier if I was in a more natural environment.*

I smile, take a deep breath, I attempt to actually radiate my inner peace outward and affect the man walking past me, going in the opposite direction. At the end of the walk I am uninspired. I was faking my peace. The walk was boring. My feet were hurting. I wish there were more trees.

Everyday we get the same instructions. "Just follow the simple directions," my teacher says.

"*Take a walk. Look around you. When your eyes rest on something, give it a name; a first generation name such as flower, paper, bug, without adding your story of . . . beautiful flower, paper that should be in a garbage can, or sweet little ladybug. Remember, this is a silent exercise.*"

Walking, Day Four: The woman in front of me is smelling the flowers, then skipping to the next patch of green where she pauses to caress the blades of grass. I think she's a total fake. *Really? She's that in love with this little patch of grass? Woman faking.* I'm annoyed with my teacher. *Follow the simple directions?* I need more. I want to yell at her: *These directions are not simple!!! Is that a sign, or is it metal, or words, or directions, or paint, or WHAT????*

Walking, Day Six: *Well fine,* I guess I can't know for sure so *woman faking* becomes *woman.* I make eye contact with a man walking who's not part of the retreat. I smile, then immediately wonder why. *Why do I always smile?*

A few days ago a woman asks me, "You always smile, are you always happy?" I am annoyed by this question, feeling totally screwed because I finally stand up in the room of 250 people so that someone can ask me any question, which I promise to answer honestly. It is meant to be an exercise in vulnerability.

Am I always happy? Of course not. What kind of question is that? Who's always happy??? So that was it.

My vulnerable confession: "No, I'm not always happy." And since then I've been questioning my smile. *Is it because I want people to like me? Because I want them to think I'm nice? Peaceful? Happy? Is it because I want them to feel comfortable or accepted themselves? How often is it sincere?*

As I walk, I make eye contact with someone else and I can't decide which way to shape the mouth of my clay-feeling face. *Follow the simple directions? THIS IS NOT SIMPLE, it's maddening! Do I smile, or not???*

Sidewalk. Woman skipping. It finally occurs to me. Without my story of needing to do it right, of wanting to be a certain type of person, of wondering about my motives and my "issues". . . without any of that, it is either *woman smiling* or *woman not smiling*. That's it.

No obsessive analysis or questioning or comparing. No right or wrong or good or bad. No manipulation. Just . . . *woman smiling*. Without the cover of my story, there is intimacy. *Woman skipping.* I take her in. *Paper on the ground. Paint on a sign.* I take it all in. I notice how having a story about each thing creates distance, as my story makes it good or bad, or something I like or don't like. Without the story I just see the woman, the paint on the sign, the paper on the ground, and it's all...so...intimate and so original, like I'm seeing it for the first time. It's all equally amazing. It's *just* what it is. Though also, it is so much more than anything I can say about it.

What is everything without my story, I wonder? Who am I? The whole world looks different. My teacher said, "No two people ever meet until they are willing to put down their story of the entire world and see the truth that stands before them." I didn't understand it then, but now it suddenly makes perfect sense.

We experience everything in life based on the story we tell about it. Good story, good experience, and vise versa. We experience life and we see people based on ourselves not on the actual situation or the person.

Cori Martinez

Avidya

"Is it true?"

– Byron Katie

Yoga teaches the concept of something called *Avidya*, which means that the story we are telling and believing about something isn't actually true. Though we are regularly afflicted by Avidya, it's hard to recognize because we don't see that something isn't true as long as we believe it is. The teachings say that Avidya is recognized more by its absence than by its presence, because in the absence of Avidya, there is profound peace.

This is big. *Every time I feel anything opposite of profound peace it's because I believe something that isn't actually true? Every time I feel anger, dissatisfaction, stress, injustice or annoyance?* Yes. That is the teaching.

As I prepare to lead my next Teacher Training, my studies seep into every aspect of my life. Through the guidance of an amazing woman named Byron Katie, I learn to ask four questions every time I feel something opposite of peace. They are designed to reveal Avidya.

- *Is it true?*
- *Can I be absolutely sure that it's true?*
- *How does it feel and how do I act when I believe this to be true?*
- *What would it be like for me if everything was the same except for my belief that this is true?*

There is a moment that haunts me, a moment I am deeply ashamed of, a night when Kalia is screaming and I believe desperately that I need her to stop.

Initially, if I ask myself in that moment, *Is it true that I need her to stop screaming?* I absolutely say yes. I say that she has been screaming for months, that we both desperately need sleep, that there is no way I can take this for another second or I am going to go crazy.

So as she screams and I believe my story that I need her to stop, *how do I feel and how do I act?* I doubt my abilities as a mother, I am a failure, I feel desperate, anxious, resentful, weak, and shamed by the heat that burns my skin. I imagine she will never stop. I imagine something is wrong with her and with me. I feel angry at Josh for not being able to make her stop, angry at him for thinking he could, and still more angry at him for giving up and leaving it ultimately to me. I scream out in anger, put Kalia roughly on the bed, and walk out of the room. I am filled with guilt and shame.

Again, according to the teachings of Avidya, if something feels anything opposite of peace, it isn't true. And I can see that this situation isn't.

After leaving Kalia in the room for a minute or two, I go back in. I am wondering, *What does every other parent know that I don't?* And then I hear my dad . . . "Babies cry." My mom has said it too, and my mother-in-law. It suddenly occurs to me there might be nothing I can do to stop her from crying. I consider that sometimes my job is not to fix everything and make it better, but just to be with whatever is arising, for both my daughter and for myself.

With this realization, I take a few deep breaths and pick her up again. I begin to rock her, feeling tethered, although so very delicately, to a place of comfort and acceptance. *This is who I am when I don't believe that I need her to stop: I am patient, loving, and I feel intimate with my child in a way I cannot be as the problem solver. This feels very peaceful.*

Is it true that I need her to stop? No. When I believe instead that I don't need her to stop, that I don't need anything to be different than it is, I am able to hold Kalia in peace for over an hour more while she continues to cry, until she finally falls asleep in my arms.

I begin to deeply understand the teachings of Avidya, to recognize it in my mind, and then to question my way out of it. Again and again I ask myself:

- *Is it true?*

- *Can I be absolutely sure that it's true?*

- *How does it feel and how do I act when I believe this to be true?*

- *What would it be like for me if everything was the same except for my belief that this is true?*

Again and again, I find in my own experience that even if I'm adamant with a yes at first, if the way I feel and act while believing something is true is anything but peaceful, I will eventually see Avidya. I will see that what I think is true is not.

Through these questions, I discover a deeper understanding of all that yoga teaches. The instructions I have studied for years, The Eight Limbs, written as guidance toward a life of union with God and experiencing inner peace, becomes so simple and obvious to me.

The instructions are:

- *Be kind*
- *Be honest*
- *Don't steal*

- *See everything and everyone as a manifestation of God*
- *Have deep gratitude without attachment to people, thoughts, or materials*
- *Clean your body inside and out*
- *Trust in the unfolding of life*
- *Be dedicated to your highest intention and disciplined in your efforts*
- *Study yourself*
- *Surrender to a higher power*
- *Do breathing exercises*
- *Do yoga postures*
- *And sit for meditation*

Though the instructions can be written simply, to live them is clearly not so simple. (At least it isn't for me.) But in my revelation of Avidya and the insight provided by asking these four questions, there is so much uncomplicated clarity. For the first time, I feel each and every one of the instructions are truly possible for me to achieve; the continued clearing out of Avidya seems to be the key.

Be kind. It doesn't happen when I believe something that isn't true. With Avidya, peace isn't a present quality. Instead, there's either an obvious or a subtle unkindness toward others and myself. The struggle to determine what actually is or isn't kind, what is or isn't necessary, or the insincerity of being kind when I really don't want to be, dissolves as Avidya dissolves. Kindness becomes natural and sincere.

Be honest, don't steal, see everything and everyone as a manifestation of God . . . it all just happens when Avidya is gone. When I realize what I think is true is not, the story that is left is always one that feels peaceful. I learn that arguing with reality is never peaceful and that trusting "what is" requires surrendering to a higher power, and I surrender.

I land in a place of feeling deeply connected to a force that is both greater than myself and an innate part of me. I haven't discovered a God who rewards and punishes or has the mind or motivation of a human being. I have discovered something much more mysterious, something entirely unfathomable; unknowable and yet deeply known within myself and everyone else I see.

The Sanskrit word for seeing everything as a manifestation of God is *Brahmacharya*. Although Brahmacharya is often taught to mean celibacy, the path of yoga I study translates this word as "Walking with God." It's an invitation to see everything as sacred, to walk through life with reverence and awe, attending to each moment as holy. Yes, even those moments we call tragic and terrible. I have found these moments have the greatest capacity for opening me up...in a way I long to open. They inspire vulnerability, compassion, empathy, humility, and they require me to fully commit to trusting and loving unconditionally.

Most people would say that miscarriage is tragic and losing a baby is terrible, yet for me it was an opportunity to feel fully and deeply connect with myself, my life, to Kalia, to Josh, to the experience of love, and the experience of loss and letting go. It was an opportunity to deepen my trust in God, or as I would have said then: in life. Through Brahmacharya, I was able to let go into my experience. Feeling it fully

allowed me to move with it and eventually through it—
or it through me—just like on my yoga mat. Without
that trust in God, life and myself, the pain would
have been so much more rigid and paralyzing. I feel
this pain each time my trust is threatened and I want
life to be different than it is.

I find that many students of yoga or other spiritual
traditions misunderstand concepts like: *Seeing God
in everything? Loving what is? Unconditional love for
everything???* They can seem quite crazy and socially
inappropriate at times. For me, the serenity prayer
made famous by Mother Theresa perfectly explains
what it means to trust in God while still actively
participating in creating our lives.

> *God grant me the serenity to accept the things
> I cannot change, the courage to change the things I
> can, and the wisdom to know the difference.*

First, ask, *What can I absolutely never change no
matter how hard I try?* The answer: Something that
has already happened or something that is already
happening. These things are absolute. They cannot

be changed no matter what.

To trust that my life is a walk with God means there's a gift in all that happens. This allows me to find serenity and unconditional love. Nothing else makes any sense. When I want Josh to be different, my mom, my dad, myself, the world, or any situation that has already come to be, or when I think anything should be different than it already is, the inner peace that comes with trusting vanishes and painful suffering ensues. *Is it true that anything should be different than it already is?* I see how believing yes hurts, and so I know it must not be true.

The thought, *I shouldn't have done that* when I already did something, brings guilt, regret, self-doubt.

They shouldn't have done that when they did, brings anger, self-righteousness, indignation and separation.

I wish it didn't happen when it did, brings defeat, envy, resentment and cynicism.

He should be more understanding when he's not, brings the feeling of being cheated.

To see my whole life as a walk with God means ending my argument with the reality of life—those things that have already happened and therefore cannot be changed without a time machine, no matter how hard I try.

I want to trust in God, in a friendly universe, in myself and in life; to trust that if it's happening it should be happening, and if it happened it should have happened, even if I can't understand why.

Yet this is not an excuse to sit passively by and not take empowered responsibility for what comes next. It's an opportunity for whatever action (or inaction) I take to be done from a place of alignment with life and what is happening, rather than from a place of resistance to life.

"I shouldn't have done that" when I did, becomes "This is what I did, and that's not who I want to be, so I'm going to apologize." Or "I'm going to learn from this and do it differently next time."

I borrowed my dad's entire retirement to open Asha Yoga and I am years late paying him back. There are many months when I barely pay the bills, and though it's hard to tell with my dad, I think he quit speaking to me for almost a year.

I sometimes become consumed by the possibility of failing, of letting everyone around me down. The shame of feeling this way as a yoga teacher and practitioner makes it worse. I think, *I should be happy and peaceful,* when I am not.

Believing I should be happy and peaceful when I'm not makes me feel like an immediate failure. It is then even harder to move. I am ashamed. I shut down and prepare to hide my struggle, to fake my smile. In that inauthenticity, that refusal to be vulnerable and real, I disengage and disconnect. I go weeks without rolling out my mat.

If, on the other hand, I choose to believe that nothing should be different—if I notice the voice of self-doubt and the desire to pull the blankets over my head and sleep for a year—and can trust that this is how it should be, then everything becomes perfect.

Right now, it should be hard. I should be struggling apparently, because I am. So many people assume and fear that accepting this reality will keep us in bed. But in my experience, I can follow that thought to, *I'm not a failure, I'm a human being. I am real, honest, complexly multi-dimensional and I am vulnerable.* In that vulnerability, I stand at the birthplace of unconditional love and connection.

Feeling the thread that unites me with my humanity and divinity, I am inspired just enough to climb out of bed and begin making breakfast for Kalia, or responding to emails, or getting on my mat. Without the weight of shame and resistance to what is, I am pulled by this thread and it is easier to move, easier to breathe. As I engage with the world, I am softer, kinder, more compassionate, less self-righteous and my smile turns out to be sincere.

The serenity of accepting and trusting the things that cannot be changed inspires the attitude from which I can most skillfully and lovingly participate in life and affect what happens next. From here, with courage, I can change the things that can be changed with love rather than anger, shame, fear or resentment. Then, I am the change I want to see already.

With willingness, I lean in, even to my regular bouts of losing trust. When suffering comes, I listen to the story my mind is telling and I just keep asking,

Is it true?

I keep observing how I react when I believe the thoughts that resist life. I see how I would behave and who I would be if instead, I trusted that there was divinity in everything.

Seven-Year Cycles

*"The extraordinary is waiting quietly beneath the
skin of all that is ordinary."*
- Mark Nepo, The Book of Awakening:
Having the Life You Want by Being
Present to the Life You Have

I'm lying in bed when Kalia tells me for the first
time, "Mom, I never want to shower with dad again.
He touched me with his penis!!!" She is appalled. She
says it with eyes wide and let's her jaw hang open at
the end of her proclamation.

It was only a week ago when Josh asked me how we were supposed to know when it was time for them to stop showering together. My response was "I don't know, I'm assuming it will just suddenly become obvious." And yep, this is OBVIOUS.

Dad touched me with his penis. I can only pray she won't repeat these words to a stranger. When I tell Josh, he is mortified. Though he has no idea what she's talking about, we can both see it's an entirely plausible (accidental) scenario.

Kalia brings it up for almost a year. "I only want to shower with you mom. I DO NOT want dad to touch me with his penis again," she says at random moments. *Oh, please God*, I pray without an ounce of spiritual connection. *Please do not let her say this in front of anyone else.*

Over a year has gone by and she's finally quit bringing up the penis story. One morning Josh gets into the shower and Kalia jumps up and says, "Can I shower with Dad?" I'm confused and unsure. We're liberal about being naked; Kalia is more liberal than we can handle. Josh and I are always having to remind her to wear underwear when she has a dress on or we have company over. Kalia will open the shower door to ask Josh questions incessantly while he's showering, so we're not worried about her seeing him naked. Just . . . *What about the whole penis thing?* And what about my philosophy that we'll know when it's time for them to stop showering together? Hadn't we gotten that signal a long time ago? "Um, I don't know," I say. "Go ask Dad."

I can hear in Josh's voice how caught off guard he is. "I guess so?" The words stumble out with a question mark. As Kalia gets into the shower I hear her say "Dad, I'm tall enough now, you don't have to pick me up to get my hair wet."

After the shower, Kalia comes back into my room and says to me, like it's the first time she's ever said anything about it, "Hey Mom, I used to not want to shower with Dad because this one time . . ." she pauses for dramatic emphasis. "This one time . . . he picked me up to get my hair wet and my toe TOUCHED his penis!!!" She looks at me like "Can you believe that???" And I can't. It's all I can do not to burst out laughing. My mind plays out the ridiculously unfortunate scenario of Josh going to jail because Kalia's toe touched his penis while he was trying to wash her hair. Josh and I decide that was their final shower together. Perfectly, Kalia also never asks again.

I have loved Josh for 14 years and I have felt loved by him for almost all of that time. Until now. Now, we seem to take each other for granted and all I hear is the list of my faults on a daily basis . . .

I don't open the windows when it's beautiful outside,

I forgot to turn the heat off again,

I didn't look through my pile of paperwork,

I left my dishes on the counter,

I didn't help enough with the household chores,

I am selfish with my time and priorities,

I don't pick up after myself,

I don't finish projects,

And on and on, until I begin to dread that he will come home for his lunch break when I am working from the house. I am so tired of not being good enough.

I see that he is right about so much of it. I wish I could be everything he wants me to be. Even more, I wish he would just want me for who I am. And if he can't, then maybe someone else will. For the first time in all these years, I feel willing to give up my marriage for the temporary passion of new and blind love. I want someone to think I'm amazing, even if only for a little while. I daydream and question. We both do.

If we separated, would we be able to work out an amicable shared custody agreement? I think so. We would both stay in Sacramento. Maybe Kalia could spend every other full week with each of us. Then every other week I would be single, and every other week I would be fully involved with homework and bedtime and frozen yogurts at Mochi.

I might have to get a roommate to share the bills and the maintenance of the house. Maybe I could rent out part of the house to someone in exchange for all the maintenance and major cleaning. They would have to like kids, but not have any because I would want the house empty and quiet during my single weeks. They would also have to be very clean, but NOT get on my case if I leave the dishes undone overnight. Maybe that could be part of the trade. They could do the dishes, put the garbage on the curb, fix the printer if it stopped working again, stop at the store to get the milk, eggs, peanut butter I forgot, and come help me if I get a flat tire on the way to work, or run out of gas, or forget my laptop and need it for a workshop I'm teaching.

Or maybe Josh would stay in the house and I could get a studio apartment. Kalia and I could share a bed. Or maybe a one bedroom—she could have the bedroom. I could make dinner for some cute guy I meet in a coffee shop during my single week and then we could make out on the couch or the living room floor with the excited, passionate anticipation that is only there with someone new and less known. We could stay up late talking about our lives, sharing all the details that make us who we are, yet sharing only what we want to, painting a picture of the person we each want the other to see, down to the perfectly constructed demonstrations of weakness and fear. We could just break it off if we saw something we didn't like.

When Kalia starts performing in school plays or dance recitals, Josh and I could both be there and be friends. Unless one of us brings a date, then how would the other behave? It makes me want to throw up to think of him sleeping with another woman, but even worse, falling in love. Or could I be happy for him? We had our time together and it was great, but now this was our time to see who else and what else our lives could be.

Kalia would be OK. Lots of kids survive their parent's divorce.

I could sleep diagonal and stack as many books as I wanted on the table next to the bed. How would I support myself? Right now Josh makes all the money. I don't want to be someone who stays married because of the kid and the financial stability. I want to be happy and madly in love. I want to spend some time with someone new, someone who doesn't know about all my issues and just thinks I'm amazing. I don't even care if it won't last; I just want it for a little while. It's been so long. I'm not sure I had enough of that before I got married. I was so young.

Am I forgetting to experience my life? To be in the moments as they are and find the beauty? I feel guilty because if I could appreciate my life for what it is, my husband for who he is, maybe I wouldn't be thinking about getting out. Maybe I'd be happy in my marriage.

Divinity in everything. Divinity in everything. Divinity in everything means . . . divinity in everything.

The truth is, some days I'm confused. There are moments when I don't know if I want to spend the rest of my life, or even the rest of my thirties, with my partner of the last 14 years. I don't know what I want to do or who I want to be.

That's what's true sometimes. When I don't fight it, there's a sweetness, a tenderness in the confusion and the doubt. I'm not here just for the result of my desperate attempts to fix everything. I'm not here just for the life I think I want, or for the painless perfect life I think I want for my daughter. I'm here to experience the life I'm living, which may include trying desperately to fix things, to make the right decision, to be a better person, to be happier and more fulfilled.

It may also include making decisions I will later regret, doing what feels wrong and failing at my efforts to be good and kind. It will undoubtedly include the soft sweet scent of forgiveness from time to time, for myself and others. It will include falling in love, infatuation, kissing a six-year-old on her chapped red mouth and hearing her tell me for the millionth time, "I love you, Mom," and falling in love again with her . . . and falling in love again with the delicate, crispy and chewy outer shell and soft buttery center of the salted caramel macarons from Ginger Elizabeth's chocolate shop on 19th and O.

I can feel the thread between this me who is a struggling wife and mother and this me who is open to it all. As I begin to trust in life once again, I feel suddenly less desperate to run.

Josh looks at me as we stand in the kitchen of the vacation rental house in Tahoe while his parents and brother and our sister-in-law and nephew and Kalia are scattered in other areas of the house and the yard.

He says, "We've been together for 14 years. I asked you to marry me. I wanted to have a baby with you.

We've been married for 10 years . . . Do you actually believe I don't think you're amazing?" And then the peace of truth washes over me as I realize, I already have everything I desperately want.

I pause to pray to God . . . please don't let me miss it.

One Letter
I Never Wrote

*"Everyone is a mirror image of yourself—your own
thinking coming back to you."*

\- Byron Katie

Dear Heather,

I think I hope you never read this. I'm not sure I
ever really liked you. I remember laughing with you,
but I also remember being annoyed by your overly
expressive, fake way of talking. *(Hmmm . . . that sounds
vaguely familiar, like my own way of talking sometimes.)*

Anyway. I never trusted you. Except that, I did. The first time I ever got a sub, I left the studio in your hands so I could go back to California for a wedding. You posted flyers for the new place you were going to teach at and gave your class schedule to every new student who came to the studio.

As a yogi, I am supposed to be OK with that. I am supposed to care more about sharing yoga with the world than business and financial matters. But as a business owner, I am supposed to stay open and pay my bills and my debts. And as a human being, I am afraid of failure.

It's been almost twelve years now that I have been in the yoga business, and some days I am still tormented by the idea that I may have to choose between business and yoga. Some days it feels like I am only pretending it's possible not to have to choose. Then, of course, some days I realize that there is no choice to be made, because they really are one in the same.

When I lived in Hawaii, I pretended to be happy that you opened your own studio around the corner, the more yoga the better. Hooray! I pretended that the thought of you didn't just completely annoy me. Except with my closest friends. They knew not to tell me if they went to "The Monkey." They could see how I literally felt crushed and betrayed, even though I would try so hard not to show it.

So many times I tried to let it go. I mean, give me a break, it was ridiculous to hold on so long. But always I secretly hoped for your failure. Just before I left Hawaii, I came to see you and I took my first class at Balancing Monkey Yoga. I can't remember the conversation, but I think we had some kind of heart to heart. It seemed that in the presence of your flesh and bones, I would always realize that you were different from the story of you I couldn't let go of. You had only always been publicly gracious and kind to me. I never knew if I could trust it because I knew my own graciousness was an act. But as I sat with you after class, I thought I had finally made peace with everything I had constructed between us and it seemed about fucking time.

After I sold the studio, I came to Hawaii and I

felt curious about you. I wondered how you were, and I didn't feel the usual resentment. It felt so good to think of you without that.

And then I heard about Max, the baby you lost eight days after he was born. I heard about your blog and I read it and . . . it was so weird how the resentment came creeping back. I expected to be so full of compassion for what you had endured, so connected to you in your pain, especially since I had lost a baby, too. But instead, I had some thought like you've made his death into an opportunity for yourself because you are so incredibly selfish. (Interesting, because my favorite piece of writing is about my own miscarriage and recovery.) For a brief moment, I hated myself for having that thought about you. The shock and shame of it was overwhelming as it threatened to take over, but I also watched it pass.

Thoughts come all the time and they aren't true. They are not a reflection of who we truly are and what we feel deep inside. They are the voice of what I often refer to as "a crazy monkey that lives inside our head," childish, self-centered, scared, confused and only able to see in black and white. It is torture to believe the thoughts that pass and to blame ourselves for their existence. In my heart, I do not see you the way I sometimes do in my mind.

Over the years, I can see how you have repeatedly shown me the parts of myself I am most ashamed of. The parts I never want anyone to see. Everything I thought about you was . . . me. You were living your life and I continued to be angry, resentful, and immature, continued to judge you and dismiss you, unable to forgive you or myself for my secret behavior toward you. But my mind believed that this was YOU I saw and not my own human self. This vicious cycle comes to an end when I am willing to admit the truth: I have never known you.

I see now that no two humans ever really meet until they are willing to put down their story of the entire world and see the truth that stands before them. I have never seen you like that. Not even close. I was always looking at the story I created of you. Once I saw that I was really seeing me, I was able to embrace this part of me and grow.

So I want to thank you. Thank you for holding that space for me for so many years. I don't know if you felt it, or if you have created your own story that is entirely different from mine, or if you have never thought twice about it. I don't know and it doesn't matter. For me you have still held that space. Thank you. And if it's been hard, I'm sorry.

With gratitude,

Cori

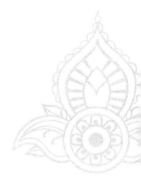

Practice

No one is with me now as I roll out my mat. Ready to roll out myself. Ready to move and breath and connect to God. There are no more doubts. There is no more hesitation. I am here to connect with divinity. I have even said it out loud. In a yoga class. "Yoga means union with God." And no one walks out the way I might have done all those years ago when I couldn't bear the word, when I refused to invite Him to my wedding, when I judged anyone who spoke His name with anything but disdain to be hypocritical and unintelligent.

Though I probably wouldn't walk out. I might not

have come back. If people don't come back to my class because I said God, I am OK with that now.

Still, I speak it gently. I ask them to just consider what it would be like to trust in something beyond their comprehension, something that connects all of humanity and makes us one? I ask how they would treat the people they meet on the street or pass on the freeway or work with or already love, but also sometimes loathe? How would they navigate through challenging times if they trust in a friendly universe with a higher goal of exploring and waking up humanity to its true nature? Waking THEM up to the highest version of themselves?

"Just what if you believed that everything was happening for you? Reflecting for you just what you needed to be a kind and compassionate being, to feel true connection, and unconditional love?"

I suggest that it might not matter whether any of it was true, because the trust alone would change their entire world.

I say it louder when I start teaching Teacher Trainings. I have to say it because I have to share it, but I do not intend to force it. There's no need. They have made it to the mat. and I know that if they keep showing up they will find out for themselves. In their own way; in their own time. I watch it happen over and over again.

I am in Sacramento, CA. I live here now. and this beautiful yoga studio is mine, as much as anything is mine. I have finally stopped name-dropping Hawaii. Mostly. I have just sold Yoga Centered.

I chant. I love it.

I drop to my knees and place my forehead on my thick black mat. I bring my hands together in a physical expression of prayer and rest them on the ground above my head.

Child's Pose.

In all my gratitude for the life I am living. I can still hear my mind... *Marriage is hard. Business is hard. Parenting is hard.*

But I know I want whatever it is. Except sometimes I forget.

I am here. on my mat, to remember.

I stretch out through my arms and spread my fingers. I turn my toes under and press my thighs up and back into Downward Dog. I move my heart space forward toward my sternum and my collarbones widen. I fill up with my breath, three dimensionally into the front, the back and the sides of my entire torso, lifting out of my shoulder joints, activating, opening, making space. I hold the shape as I exhale, surrender and smile.

I begin to move and breathe. I listen deeply. I might find resistance, irritation, sadness, boredom, rigidity . . . I notice each thing as it is and I move with it for a while. Until eventually I begin to move through it. Or does it move through me? I'm not sure. But as I unfold, unravel, let go, breathe in and breathe out, whatever I find to be holding me back, to be moving me away from myself and from God, dissolves into a whisper that glides from my lips as hello and thank you. Each movement becomes a prayer. An expression of my own divinity and my desire to know this God inside of me and everyone else I will ever know.

Today I repeat silently with each breath, *divinity in everything, divinity in everything.*

I am not sure if my marriage is going to make it.

Being a Yoga Teacher
Part Two

"I saw that we're all doing the best we can. This is how a lifetime of humility begins."

— Byron Katie

Over the past 14 years, I have practiced yoga in order to sweat and to do what my friends were doing. I've worn $120 yoga pants, spent that same amount on a sticky mat, drank martinis after a yoga class, eaten pork belly, been a hypocrite, judged myself and others, and yelled at my husband, my daughter, and my mother.

I've wanted bigger classes; I've modeled for yoga photo shoots showing off my most impressive yoga postures, dyed my hair, been greedy, selfish, depressed and lost. I've done all of these things while simultaneously discovering a level of compassion for myself and others, which allows me to stop judging and deeply connect.

I've made peace with the loss of a baby, fallen in love with the challenges of motherhood and marriage, as well as seen the joys more clearly. I've forgiven myself for not always being who I hope to be. And I have met God . . . in myself, in the members of my family, my friends, students, strangers I pass on the street, and in the general, yet wondrous, circumstances of life.

People practice yoga today for many reasons, and sometimes it looks from the outside as if they aren't doing "real yoga." In fact, it often looks this way from the inside too, as we judge ourselves. And sometimes we are practicing and have no idea or interest in how deeply we're going. But I believe that if we're practicing, and we're doing the best we can with what we have and what we know, we're doing "real yoga," and headed inward to something amazing. I also believe that we all do the best we can in every moment, whether we know it or not and whether others believe it or not. I think if we had the capacity to do better, we would, and, in time, we will.

Finding real yoga on the cover of Yoga Journal magazine, at a gym, in an expensive outfit, without breathwork or meditation, before binging on food or alcohol or after a cup of coffee doesn't mean there aren't deeper places to go and that we're not headed straight there. (And it doesn't mean that kind of practice is what I teach or prefer or promote.)

When I was practicing to sweat, I brought space heaters into the room when I taught. When my goal was to do a handstand, I taught core work, Plank, upper backbends, shoulder openers, and I talked about courage and fear. When I saw myself as selfish and practiced to cultivate generosity, I taught less about alignment and more about breath. When my body and heart needed to heal, the classes I taught were slower and softer. My teaching has always moved in alignment with my practice and my life.

These days I practice for physical, mental and spiritual connection. My teaching is precise, detailed, and focused in the body and mind while also being bigger than a yoga pose. I challenge myself to be vulnerable. I invite students to look inward, dig deep, and laugh or cry.

I take yoga both lightly and very sincerely, knowing that it's simultaneously my entire life and such a small part of my entire life. It is both the background of everything I do and a distant object that belongs to others, depending on the moment, depending on the time and place.

I once read in Deborah Adele's book *Yama and Niyama* that she had a friend who said her greatest fear was ending up in a room with everyone she knew all at once and not knowing who to be.

I'm married to a man who's never stepped foot in a yoga studio except to make repairs and never opened a yoga magazine except to look for Kathryn Budig's latest nude ToeSox ad. I don't have an altar in my house; I do have a TV, and I have used it to watch "The Bachelor!!!"

Sometimes this life makes my yoga life seem miles away, possibly even belonging to someone else. Then I remember that Kalia spends every single night listening to a guided Yoga Nidra meditation for kids before bed. When things get tense, we both calm ourselves with deep breathing. I try all the time to have an open mind, an open heart and to be present with her.

My yoga mat lives behind the couch in the living room and I unroll it regularly in front of the fireplace or by the sliding glass door in my bedroom. I sit regularly for meditation in my car, using a timer on my phone. When I open my eyes I see a bird and I hear the wind and the rustle of trees so clearly that I am nearly always struck with awe.

There are times when every ordinary, mundane thing feels sacred. That's when yoga seems to be the backdrop for everything I do. Vacillating back and forth between a life where I worry I'm an imposter for teaching yoga because it feels so distant and a life where I realize it's all yoga and that distance isn't possible, is sometimes confusing. Sometimes heart wrenching. But I find it to be a beautiful part of going deeper.

Despite having felt like a phony as a teacher when I couldn't live up to my own ideas of what a yogi should be, making me feel like a failure, a hypocrite, or a fraud, this experience, over time, has led me to a freedom that has been instrumental in my ability to support others in finding their own freedom.

After I yell at Josh, numb myself with TV, gossip about a friend, or get defensive with a family member, I feel less self-righteous and judgmental of others for doing the same. I feel more compassionate, vulnerable, and clear about who I want to be.

I've learned that the role of a yoga teacher is not to be perfect in the ways one might think. That it's important I see my own humanness within the journey and then the humanness of others.

Being human means I will sometimes fail, I will sometimes react, I will sometimes disconnect, disengage, get defensive, get angry, hurt, self-righteous, self-centered, and narrow-minded . . . Yes, even as a yoga teacher! Opening to the possibility that I am imperfectly perfect allows me to soften, to feel lighter, and to forgive myself and others when I stumble.

As a teacher, I learn and then I share my experience. I understand, because I've been there myself. I tell students inquiring as to whether they're ready to teach, "If you are alive and paying attention to your life, then you have something to offer. Breathe in the fear and self-doubt that may arise, feel it completely, and then move on. If you want to teach, just do it. Don't let fear and self-doubt hold you back."

Meeting myself where I am allows me to meet others where they are, too. That is a beautiful gift.

Cori Martinez

Working It Out
With My Dad

"I came to see that the world is always as it should be, whether I opposed it or not. And I came to embrace reality with all my heart. I love the world, without any conditions."
– Byron Katie

I'm sitting on a barstool in my kitchen when my grandfather calls. When he starts talking, I start to pace. Then my knees get weak. I lower to the ground in slow motion and I think I stop breathing. I don't know why. Is it because that's how a daughter is supposed to react when she finds out her dad is in the hospital? Or is it because he had gone in four days ago, and finding out now was heartbreaking proof of the non-existent relationship between us?

Only my grandfather has known that he's been in the hospital. My dad doesn't want anyone else to know, so he makes my grandfather promise not to tell me. "But he doesn't sound good," says my grandfather. Despite my dad's wishes, he is telling me anyway.

My dad is at the VA hospital in Fresno, a three-hour drive from my house. I tell my grandfather I'll go there right away. It's something about his heart, but my dad didn't make a big deal of things like this, so there is no way of knowing the severity by talking to him.

I am extra aware of my own heartbeat, and I feel a little light-headed, but I am dry eyed when I call Josh. Until he says hello and I attempt to speak. Then I start to cry. Is he OK? "I don't know." What happened? "I don't know." Did you call the hospital? "No."

When I had my miscarriage my dad drove five hours to see me, without calling to say he was coming.

It annoyed me then. I didn't want him there. I didn't have it in me to play the part of his daughter, to pretend we had a relationship, to be interested in what he had to say even if I wasn't interested.

As I stand in the shower getting ready to go see him in the hospital I wonder, *Does he feel the same way? Is that why he doesn't want me to know?* I guess I thought that even though I didn't have a relationship with him, as the parent, he had one with me that he just didn't know how to express. But now I begin to wonder.

When he had come to see me after my miscarriage, I felt like his visit was totally selfish. He should have called; he should have asked what I wanted. Now, as hot water streams over my head and body, I understand. I know he doesn't want me to come to the hospital, but I don't care. I'm not doing it for him. I'm doing it for me. Even if it is selfish, I need to do it.

I get dressed and pack my bags. Josh comes home, gives me directions and loads up my car.

Just before I leave the house, I look at the family photo wall I completed just days ago. It includes my mom, because I knew if it didn't, her feelings would be hurt. I had specifically searched for photos of her and was relieved to locate the one of her and Kalia from the mall. It includes Josh's mom, dad, brother, our sister-in-law and nephew because of a photo shoot Josh's mom had arranged. There are two pictures from our wedding, one of which I had purposefully picked because it includes Bob. And there are three blank frames waiting for a picture of my niece, my nephew and Kalia's best friend, Grace. I realize as I stand there that it hadn't even occurred to me to put a picture of my dad on the wall.

The guy at the information center near the hospital entrance says my dad is on the fifth floor. I take the elevator up and find the nurses' station. A nurse points down a long hallway toward a door with a window and says, "Go through that door and then you'll have to call to be let into the next room." I walk down the hallway and stop at the door with the window. I stare at the sign, which reads: ICU Family Waiting Area.

Up until this moment I've had no idea whether

he'd had a massive heart attack or a case of heartburn. Staring at this sign, I realize for the first time . . . it definitely isn't heartburn. I feel relief that I have come. I also begin to play a story in my head of how happy my dad will be to see me, how grateful he will be that I am here with him. Although I'm scared of his condition, another small part of me feels excitement for this chance to connect.

When I get to his room he's sleeping. There are tubes taped to his arm and a monitor tracking his heart. He looks grey. And old.

He wakes up after only a few seconds, and he smiles. "Somebody is in trouble," he says, referring to my grandfather. But his smile has me convinced that my story stands a chance; that he is actually, secretly, glad I am here.

Even when I tell him "DAD!!! You have to tell me if you're in the hospital. I have a right to know," and he responds, "No, I don't. It's none of your business and I have a right for you not to know," I still believe he is just being stubborn and that this is not a reflection of his true feelings.

Apparently his body had completely swollen up and he was having trouble breathing, so he drove himself to the nearest VA hospital, which was two hours away from his house. The doctors found his heart to be pumping twice as fast as it should be. Over the past four days, they had drained three gallons of excess water from his body and have not been able to slow his heart. They are calling it congestive heart failure.

He spends seven days in the ICU and I am there for the two in the middle. After the first day, there is nothing more to talk about. We sit watching TV while I become increasingly disappointed that he won't change his mind and just be happy I am there. He won't agree that being in the hospital is something I should know about. He doesn't call to tell me when he is released. It takes me some time to let the disappointment and anger subside.

I tell my mom, he could be dead lying in his house for weeks and nobody would know. Nobody is checking in on him.

"That's just the way he'd want it," she says.

And though at first I can't possibly believe that it's true, though my mind screams that it shouldn't be this way, that it's not fair to me or to my daughter . . . if I sit in silence long enough, I am able to trust in the reality of what is.

I am able to see that, in my anger, there is beauty born of love for my dad. It is born of a desire to be there for him and with him. In my resistance there is opportunity for my own growth and awakening. *Can I allow my dad to be who he is, and love him anyway? Can I allow myself to be disappointed and then forgive us both?*

Can I see all the ways in which I don't allow my own self to be looked after and supported, all the ways in which I too am stubborn and impenetrable, and feel the closeness to my dad in these shared qualities?

Can I see that what I resist in him is only a reflection of what I resist within me?

When I sit in silence, I see God in all of it, and the answer is yes, yes, and yes.

The answer to all of life is yes.

Cori Martinez

Mystery

"Walk slowly into the mystery."

– Danna Faulds

The first several times I ask myself the question . . . *Where is she getting this from?* I am completely oblivious to the possibility that she is getting it all from Josh and me.

I am looking at her across a field of grass, noticing the way she stands with both legs straight, one hand on her jutting out hip, head tilted slightly to the side as she watches something intently. I watch her for almost a full minute before I catch a glimpse of my own legs, and my eyes follow up my hips to my arms. I see in my own body the mirror image of Kalia's stance in that very moment, my head also tipping slightly to the side. I had never noticed how I stood, but in this moment it feels so comfortable and familiar that I know it is a way I often stand. And I see that it is now the way Kalia stands. I thought . . . *She does what I do.*

By age six she already knows much more than me, in her world. I remember being this way with my mom. As a child, as a teenager, and even now as an adult, I always think I know more than my mom. It drives my mom crazy, which I finally understand. I tell Kalia, "You are six. I am 32. Who do you think knows more???" She says "It's been longer since you were in school, so I think I do," and she means it completely.

As she sits at the counter refusing to admit that she misspoke, insisting instead that Josh and I both heard her incorrectly, over a thing so small I can't even remember it now, I see her eyes fill with tears and desperate determination, and I can relate. She is desperate not to have made a mistake.

She has a hard time saying she's sorry. Like me. I will often defend myself tirelessly before apologizing, as if my convincing the other person that I didn't actually do anything wrong will improve my standing in their eyes (and therefore in my own). Every yoga teacher is familiar with the infamous quote by Gandhi, "You must be the change you wish to see in the world." In an effort to be a good teacher, I apologize to Kalia so as to lead by example, forgetting that she can see and hear the way Josh and I stubbornly refuse to say we're sorry to each other.

One day, I am sitting calmly at the kitchen counter eating breakfast and Kalia is putting on a pair of socks. She stands up and immediately begins to have a break down. Stomping her foot and flinging her arms, she shouts, "IT'S NOT COMFORTABLE!!" I know what the problem is. She's incredibly sensitive to the seam at the toe of her socks. This was a regular occurrence, and this day I handled it by slamming my hand down on the counter and shouting right back at her, "KALIA! YOU DO NOT NEED TO GET SO UPSET OVER ONE LITTLE THING! CALM DOWN!"

For so long I have heard the words: "You must be the change you want to see in the world," and I generically wanted peace and kindness and knew that it was within my power to bring those things to the world by living it in my own life. But since the moment Kalia was born, she has been the one to show me, in sometimes-painful detail, exactly how to do this.

With her defensive insistence, her pained resistance, her desperate tears, and her temper tantrums, she shows me and inspires me more than likely anyone else in the world can. I want peace for her even more than I want it for the entire world.

So I do whatever I think *she* should do: I admit that I don't know everything. I ask my own mother for advice. I tell Josh that I'm sorry. I take a deep breath and notice the words I want to scream at her, then I whisper them to myself instead ... *I do not need to get so upset over one little thing. Calm down.*

I live the change I want to see in the world by

living the advice I have for my daughter. As I watch her, it is clear that "Do as I say, not as I do" isn't an option. No matter what I say, *Kalia does what I do.* She is the clearest possible reflection of me, showing me constantly who I am. My love for her, my intense desire for her happiness and freedom, invites me to be vulnerable and comfortable with uncertainty, to be emotionally exposed, to risk failure, to admit not knowing, and to love myself and others no matter what.

After a miscarriage, many people point out that *I can try again.* But I don't want to. I have come to see my second pregnancy as such a beautiful gift of love and loss and realization that it feels like more than enough. My work building a new yoga studio, a new community for myself in Sacramento, along with the family community I had come back for, and Kalia and Josh ... It is all so deeply satisfying and consuming that I don't want to miss any of it by adding more.

Then, I am sitting in my mother-in-law's kitchen with her and my sister-in-law, Christina. My mother-in-law pours a glass of champagne for each of us, just because, and Christina declines.

My mother-in-law's eyes light up, her voice gets a little quieter, and she already has a knowing smile when she asks Christina, "Are you pregnant?" She is.

I don't expect to barely be able to get the words out. I don't expect it to be so hard to smile. "Congratulations," I say. "I'll be right back." I didn't expect to start crying uncontrollably, but the moment I am out of earshot that's exactly what happens.

That night I cry to Josh and he says to me for the first time, "I have always wanted us to try again, but I have never wanted to pressure you."

Fear begins to well up inside of me and I hear a whisper of *no*. I listen.

No. I don't want another baby; I only want the baby I never got to have. I feel the pain of resisting reality, of arguing with God and life about what cannot be changed.

No. No. No. I can't risk it. No. I'm too afraid. And for the first time I begin to question whether I have truly found peace through healing or if I have instead built a sheath of steel armor that has been protecting me from still very present pain.

A few days later, on our tenth wedding anniversary, Josh tells me that he just can't move forward without making one final case for having another baby. He asks me to listen, and then he promises to accept my decision, whatever it is. I begin to imagine our life with another child. Maybe more full, more rewarding, more complete. And then we start trying to get pregnant.

Two months later I don't start my period. But the pregnancy test shows negative.

Multiple weeks pass and I still don't start my period. I begin to read stories on the Internet about all the women who've had babies while never showing positive, even with a blood test. I am convinced I'm one of those women, but at the same time I'm afraid to get my hopes up.

One day while lying on my yoga mat I realize that in my fear, in the wearing of my armor of self-preservation, I am missing the opportunity of love. Because regardless of how the future is going to unfold, it is my choice right now to feel love, or to keep myself from feeling it.

In this moment it seems an opportunity so obviously worth the risk. My heart cracks open and I fall quickly and deeply in love with a baby growing inside of me.

And after eight weeks I start to bleed.

I don't think it's a miscarriage. I have taken several more home pregnancy tests and just taken a blood test. All results say I am not pregnant.

That day I decide, once again, that what I have is enough. After just celebrating his 39th birthday, Josh also begins to feel like he may not be up for having another baby at this point. We stop trying to get pregnant again.

I don't know. Did healing happen in finally letting go of fear, in my willingness to feel love and possibly loss once again? Or is the fear inside me still, now even more cleverly masked? Can I only be willing to risk a limited number of times before I must once again begin to protect myself?

I don't know. And I don't need to.

I know of the existence of something unfathomable, impenetrable, and this knowledge is as unexplainable as the thing I know, the thing I call God. And if God, this unexplainable force, is at the heart of my life, of all life, then how can I expect to understand the workings of any life fully?

Yes, my mind wants answers. It questions, assumes, guesses, analyzes, hypothesizes, and questions again and again, looking for security and solutions. *What do my actions prove about me and what do other's actions prove about them? Is it my fault or is it their fault? Is it right or wrong? Good or bad? What is the solution?* But a man of great intelligence has said,

"We cannot solve a problem with the same mind that created it." Thank you Albert Einstein, my heart can see this to be true. It can see another way to be in the world.

Anchored in divinity, I can cherish the inexplicable dimensions of life. I can give up on the idea that I will ever put all the pieces together, and I can respect the mystery and the miracle. I can acknowledge that settling on an answer limits the majesty of the question and the experience.

I can choose to let the mystery be ever so much more than enough.

Albert Einstein also wrote, "The fairest thing we can experience is the mysterious." He claimed in his work, *The World as I See It*, "It was the experience of mystery that engendered religion. A knowledge of the existence of something we cannot penetrate, of the manifestations of the profoundest reason and the most radiant beauty, which are only accessible to our reason in their most elementary forms."

Einstein believed that the human qualities we humans so often give to God, "A God who rewards and punishes his creatures, or has a will of the type of which we are conscious of in ourselves, are notions for the fears or absurd egoism of feeble souls." Instead he chooses mystery. He says, "Enough for me the mystery of the eternity of life, and the inkling of the marvelous structure of reality, together with the single-hearted endeavor to comprehend a portion, be it never so tiny, of the reason that manifests itself in nature."

In this I find peace. Although my mind may never

find the answers that it seeks, it is more than enough to say yes to living and trusting in the mystery.

Not needing to know, I can willingly, humbly, curiously follow the mystery wherever it leads me. All the while recognizing the power of God within me to create the world of my dreams.

We all can.

Cori Martinez

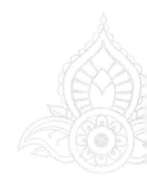

Practice

Is it true?

Some days it is still my physical practice that jostles my mind from it's deeply automated perceptions, and wakes me up to a greater truth.

Today I lie down on my mat and bend my knees. I bring the bottoms of my feet together and allow my knees to drop out to the sides. It's a vulnerable position. My groin, belly, heart—wide open. But somehow there is safety on the mat and I am not uncomfortable with the shape. I am grateful. Yet sad. I lay one hand over my belly and one hand over my heart and feel movement flowing through. Belly rising, chest rising, then falling, rising then falling.

The day has been a challenge.

Belly rising, chest rising, falling, rising, falling.

I bring my knees together and hug them into my chest. Then I reach my arms out to the sides and lower both knees to the right. My spine rotates, wringing out the tension in my back. I breathe deeply into my whole torso: front, side, and back expanding with each inhale, letting go with each exhale. After several minutes I twist to the other side and keep breathing deeply, reaching beyond the perimeter of my physical body with the breath, reaching to connect to something larger than my own individual life.

Today there is no music.

There is just the whisper of my breath, the noise outside, and the nagging voice in my mind.

I am tempted to get up. To walk away from my mat. It seems too hard to stay. But then I wonder, is it harder to stay or harder to keep living in resistance to life?

I unwind from the twist, and pause.

Belly rising, chest rising, falling, rising, falling.

I stay. I move into a seated forward bend, still heavy. Until finally, I notice that the extra weight brings me deeper into my forward bend and feels good on my hamstrings. I smile ever so slightly as I realize the pleasure in carrying my burden today, and I watch my story transform. It really is OK. I really am OK.

As I close my practice, hands in prayer at the center of my chest, head bowing slightly toward my fingertips, there is a glimmer of trust that everything is just as it should be, that everything is right.

I whisper. . . Namaste.

Cori Martinez

Afterword

"When they attack you and you notice that you love them with all your heart, your work is done."

— Byron Katie

I sit writing the final pages of this book a few weeks after 20-year-old Adam Lanza fatally shot twenty children and six adult staff members in a mass murder at Sandy Hook Elementary School.

I have been teaching yoga now for 14 years.

When I heard about the shootings, and watched the images, and read the stories, my stomach churned. I had just come from leading an Advanced Yoga Study and Teacher Training Retreat where we deeply explored the concept of Brahmacharya, seeing divinity in everything, seeing the light in everything. *Could I do that here? Could anyone?*

First, I sat with my humanity, with the anger, the sadness, and the repulsion that came.

But I was also waiting . . .

All things.

I know how crazy this may sound, but as I felt my own heart opening up for the children and their families, as I heard people express again and again how they were hugging their children tighter, vowing not to take life for granted, praying and sending love to strangers, I saw this as a gift these children gave to millions. The longer I sat acknowledging the light, the less I saw tragedy.

"Tragedy," for me, is a word that cannot hold the fullness of what I saw: Loss *and* gain. Hearts breaking *and* hearts opening. And the less I called it a tragedy in my own mind, the more love I felt in my own heart, the more my trust in the divinity of all things was restored.

It seemed to me I could honor these children by acknowledging the gift of love they were giving the world. It seemed I could honor them more by not calling their death a tragedy. The resistance I felt was only to the possibility that we would all be so busy calling it a tragedy, arguing about gun laws and politics, and screaming about the horror, that we wouldn't allow ourselves to feel the reminder to love more, care more, show it more, and say it more. *And that we wouldn't pause to see how our anger would cause more of the pain and suffering that created this event in the first place.*

From my experience of losing a baby, I know that we often need to be in pain and anger and other stages of grief—we need to see our experience as tragic and terrible with no possibility of light—to feel the depth and breadth of our sorrow so that our wounds may heal. I get that one hundred percent. That is the human experience. It's part of what I believe we're here for, to feel whatever comes up. Fully.

But I also believe that we are all connected, and that if *I* don't need to be in that stage, I can hold a space of trust in the universe, of love and light in all things, and that will contribute to another human being's process of moving through those stages and eventually finding peace.

It is from this spirit that I expressed myself on Facebook soon after the shooting, calling to anyone who may be able to hold this space with me and see the light, the gift, and the opportunity to open our hearts and honor these kids for reminding us. People were saying, "Now is a time to love our children, to feel gratitude for our lives," and I was asking, *What reminded us to do that?* Those kids and, dare I say, that gunman.

So in a fairly brief post I proposed that *in that reminder* we were given a gift and that we could honor those kids by accepting it with grace and using it for good, by opening our hearts and loving more so that we could do our part to contribute peace to the situation rather than outrage.

This was much appreciated by many. The post reached out to thousands and there were some very beautiful expressions of gratitude. *And it was not at all appreciated by others.* People in the larger yoga community also called me vile, nuts, a sick individual, a poor leader, and an asshole.

For clarity, I am not saying that the death and shooting was the gift. I am saying that the resulting outpouring of love and compassion for strangers, the increased connection with our own families and lives, the chance to find compassion for those we are so quick to hate (like the gunman, yes, and also the people we disagree with in the world: the people who cut us off on the freeway, the people who treat us poorly, the people who call us vile). *The opportunity to increase our love and compassion is what I am calling the gift.*

But, yes, I am also saying that given this gift, the death and shooting becomes bigger than tragedy for me. What if we were talking about a child who was killed by a drunk driver, and that child's heart was donated to another dying kid, and because of one child's death another was able to live? This is a gift, which resulted from death, more easily seen. The picture is bigger than a tragic drunk driving accident.

What if the child who lived went on to cure cancer? Or what if he went on to be a murderer? I am saying the death of the child who donated his heart is honored more when the child who lives tries to do something good with his life.

What if the boy who was given the heart could only see tragedy in how he got the heart? Do you think he would feel gratitude for his life? Or would he feel guilt? Which do you think is going to inspire him more to do something good with his life, his gratitude for the chance to live or his guilt for why he is able to live?

For me, seeing beyond the tragedy toward the possibility for greater connection, personal responsibility and compassion, inspires me to act from love and be the change I want so much to see in the world. For me, this is not about *looking on the bright side*. This is about seeing the light in the dark, about seeing the light in all things (or trusting that it's there when I can't see it) so that I may change the world by living in peace.

Martin Luther King Jr. said it this way: "Darkness cannot drive out darkness, only light can do that. Hate cannot drive out hate, only love can do that."

Do I wish there wasn't violence in the world? Of course. And once it becomes something that cannot be changed because it has already happened, my practice is to trust in the light and the divinity and to let that light guide my inner state and my actions in an effort to keep it from happening again.

The antidote to violence cannot possibly be violence. How many ways do I increase the violence I see in the world when I stand in judgment and separation? From that distance, it is easy for me to interpose my own passive forms of violence in the world, creating pain that is more emotional. Many of us may believe that passive violence such as religious or political intolerance, harsh words, name-calling, insults, dishonest communication, angry looks, eye rolling, manipulation, interrupting, putting down, ostracizing, or humiliating another person is far less destructive than physical brutality or murder, but Gandhi taught that passive violence is even more insidious than physical violence. He taught that passive violence generates anger and defensiveness in the victim, which is the fuel for all physical violence in the world.

How much fuel have I given to the physical violence in the world? That is what I can begin to change.

One of my students, who is a passionate and dedicated social worker, messaged me personally in response to my post about the shooting. She was struggling with a belief that as outrage turns to purpose, good things can happen.

I respectfully disagree.

I have heard a version of this hundreds of times. I have worked very closely with many yoga students who believe desperately that anger and outrage are needed to inspire positive action . . . and after in-depth inquiry and self-study, I have seen most of them realize for themselves that, in fact, they are not.

The negative comments made on my post,

calling me vile, sick, an asshole, etc. are an example of violence masquerading as love, and it only tears us apart. These people were angry with me because they believed I was disrespecting the families in pain and they likely believed they were doing good to defend those families and berate me. Many others were angry about politics, gun laws, the media, the failings of society, and so on. Much of this anger was masquerading as love for those kids and those families. But all of this anger was only causing more anger. It was fueling the fire in ways we can't even begin to track.

But if outrage cannot lead to good, then how is there a gift in the outrage of the gunman? Without the love *there is no gift,* there is only tragedy. The love *is* the light, the divinity, and the only way there can be a gift.

When I first read the harsh words directed at me, my reactions vacillated between defensive, hurt, and pissed off. Only because I trusted there was light in those words and in that experience for me, was I able to sit with my reactions, honor and acknowledge them by seeking support and discourse with friends, without responding, until I could do so with a clear and open heart.

It was my trust in that light, not the harsh words, which showed me one more time that everything is divine, and allowed me to continue acting in a way I can be proud of. But the hardest time to trust in that light is in the face of violence, anger, or outrage, which is why actions that come from those places are never as effective when the goal is love. Emotional violence is the fuel for physical violence.

The overwhelming response to the shooting was hurt, anger, and repulsion. The rare response was to use the pain as an incubator for compassion and intention toward healing, learning, and serving.

If we want to see more love in the world, let's NOT hope the world gets angry. Let's hope that we can start loving ourselves and our neighbors so much that we start treating everyone better, and *that* reaches out endlessly.

And let us begin by doing it ourselves.

Love everywhere, love unconditionally, and love

everything.

That is how I open my heart, how I meet the best version of myself, how I connect with humanity, and with God. That is my practice and my message.

This, in fact, is the yogic message of my time. As yoga teachers, we theme classes about connection, about opening our hearts, about loving what is. We say *Namaste* at the end of every yoga class, meaning, "the divine light within me recognizes the divine light in you, and we acknowledge we are one." We post about it on Facebook, write blogs about it and books. But all of it is meaningless if we aren't willing to apply it when it's hard, when it seems like it can't possibly hold up. Those are the moments that count and that make all the difference in the world.

Can we look into the face of violence and make space in our heart for love?

Can we sit with pain and discomfort without calling it bad and pushing it away?

Can we climb down from our tower of knowing what's right and how things should definitely be, and not be, and make space for a force that is bigger than our individual story?

Can we be open to receive a gift in an unrecognizable form?

Can we be willing to take personal responsibility for what we see in the world, to stop pointing the finger outward and instead look within, even when the whole world agrees the problem is *someone else*?

Is any of this easy? Absolutely not.

But in my experience it is even harder to see darkness, to blame others, to be powerless, and to be separate.

We have believed we are separate long enough. If we can endure the challenge of that experience, we certainly have the capacity to love, to trust, to see God everywhere. We can truly connect to each other, to God and to ourselves as God.

Therein lies the practice.

Chronology
(2006–2011)

I chanted Om. But just once. I had to. Everyone else was. Began to ponder. Yoga means Union. Union with God. Or higher power. Our true nature. New age mumbo-jumbo. Wait a minute. Is that new? Is that God? I Om'ed more. It just happened. Began to share. Started a blog. Something to offer? I was confident. And I wasn't. I themed classes. All for me. I needed it. To hear it. I felt pressure. I wasn't perfect. Wanted to be. Daycare for Kalia. Was that OK? Shopped at Co-op. Cooked with mother-in-law. Skipped teacher meetings. Made some friends. AMK and Julia.

243

Wanted another baby. Finally got pregnant. We told Kalia. She thought boy. She was sure. We told everyone. I started spotting. Called the doctor. Not to worry. Had an ultrasound. Saw the baby. Heart wasn't beating. Doctor said sorry. Handed me Kleenex. He felt bad. I just cried. Josh cried too. This was rare. I had options. Could have D&C. Take some pills. Or just wait. I just waited. Lying in bed. I kept crying. I wanted to. I wanted sadness. Talked to friends. Heard their stories. I never knew. It finally happened. So much blood. I was ready. I realized something. This was it. It always was. Never a toddler. Never a teen. No other future. Always only this. I told Kalia. In her bed. She was crying. I was silent. She didn't understand. I let her. I watched her. I loved her. I felt something. Something like God. Could've tried again. But we didn't.

Opened Asha Yoga. Sold Yoga Centered. Lived in Sacramento. 3 years now. I just noticed. Marriage was hard. Business was hard. Parenting was hard. Found four questions. Is it true? Ten-day intensive. Intensive self-inquiry. Raised my hand. I was ready. I wanted freedom. She had noticed. "You always smile." She asked me. "You're always happy?" I was irritated. I got screwed. Who's always happy? A wasted question. I still smiled. But smiling sucked. I questioned smiling. I questioned happy. And then I noticed. It was simple. A woman smiling. I didn't analyze. I felt free. Thanks for asking. I kept noticing. She wanted love. She wanted respect. She wanted control. She was me. And she wasn't. A woman sitting. A woman standing. A woman smiling. So very simple. It was intimate. And also separate. Still felt free.

Ten years teaching. I said it. I said God. It wasn't bad. No one left. Are you uncomfortable? Some said yes. But that changed. We opened up. We opened together. We understood God. It was different. God was different. Not for everyone. It was OK. I spoke mumbo-jumbo. New-age crap. I loved it. I loved God. Loved my life. Saw the sacred. In the ordinary. Smiled at Ego. Woman smiling again. It was sweet. I still complained. It was perfect. I was perfect. But not always. Started training teachers. Was I qualified? Some said yes. Not at first. Gotta start somewhere.

Had no money. Barely paid bills. The owner again. And dead broke. So I say. Had a house. I ate organic. I still traveled. Josh did well. He was stressed. We watched TV. I admit it. We drank martinis. Not very often.

Kalia started Kindergarten. A perfect school. A Montessori charter. She hated sitting. Crisscross apple sauce. "Jobs" were boring. Boring, boring, boring. This was life. Now I understand. Could be boring. Could be hard. Could be beautiful. Up to me. A friendly universe. If I trusted. A friendly God. Same difference now. I started chanting. Despite my mom. Om, Jai Ganesha. There was Caroline. (Not her real name). Yoga Teacher Trainee. She didn't chant. I could relate. Then she did. My heart skipped. We found God. She and I. She didn't know. But I did. He wasn't upstairs. Wasn't a "he." It was this. What we felt. When we chanted. I tread lightly. I say "Universe." I say . . . "Maybe." Consider, what if?

Life is perfect. I might notice. I might not. Might see fighting. Might doubt myself. Take things personally. That's OK too. New secret treasure. I am grateful. Thank you, Mom. Thank you, Josh. Thank you, Kalia. All my family. All my friends. Thank you, students. Across the country. Thank you, teachers. Thank you, God.

About the Author

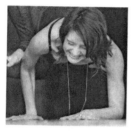 Cori Martinez teaches self-inquiry and yoga retreats, yoga teacher trainings, and yoga workshops across the country. She writes for prominent yoga and wellness websites such as MindBodyGreen, elephant journal, and YOGANONYMOUS, and also writes her own successful blog, Thread of Spirit. She is a devoted wife and mother, and the founder of Asha Yoga in Sacramento, CA.

Cori's teaching style is to support movement both on the mat and through life with honesty, skill, and grace. As a teacher, she is known for inspiring her students to be totally honest with themselves and their practice, for her mastery at conveying a clear understanding of how the body works, and for her ability to create an environment where students can connect to the highest version of themselves, their life, and the divine.

Praise for Workshops, Retreats and Training with Cori Martinez

"Cori Martinez brings an element of 'realness' to her teaching with honesty, candor and humor."
– Amanda Tomac

"Cori Martinez is truly an expert and master teacher. She presents the subject of yoga with skill, clarity, passion, and wisdom." – Jennifer Varley

"Cori's inspiring strength and enthusiasm helped me find a deeper understanding both physically and spiritually. This led to a freedom in myself I had never known, but always wished for." – Robin Mordecai

"Cori has a knowledge of the body that is rare in the yoga world." – Kate McKinney

"My heart feels so full of love, respect and gratitude. Training with Cori was truly an amazing experience."
– Laura Walcott

---

www.ashayoga.com • www.corimartinez.com